T0175197

POCKET GUIDE FOR THE
ASSESSMENT AND TREATMENT OF EATING DISORDERS

Copyright © 2019 American Psychiatric Association Publishing

ALL RIGHTS RESERVED

First Edition
Manufactured in the United States of America on acid-free paper
22   21   20   19   18   5   4   3   2   1

American Psychiatric Association Publishing
800 Maine Avenue SW
Suite 900
Washington, DC 20024-2812
www.appi.org

Library of Congress Cataloging-in-Publication Data
Names: Lock, James, editor. | American Psychiatric Association, issuing body.
Title: Pocket guide for the assessment and treatment of eating disorders / edited by James Lock.
Description: First edition. | Washington, D.C. : American Psychiatric Association Publishing, [2019] | Includes bibliographical references and index.
Identifiers: LCCN 2018034927 (print) | LCCN 2018035425 (ebook) | ISBN 9781615372157 (ebook) | ISBN 9781615371563 (paperback : alk. paper)
Subjects: | MESH: Feeding and Eating Disorders—diagnosis | Feeding and Eating Disorders—therapy | Handbooks
Classification: LCC RC552.E18 (ebook) | LCC RC552.E18 (print) | NLM WM 34 | DDC 616.85/26—dc23
LC record available at https://lccn.loc.gov/2018034927

British Library Cataloguing in Publication Data
A CIP record is available from the British Library.

Contents

Contributors

Sarah Adler, Psy.D.
Clinical Assistant Professor, Department of Psychiatry and Behavioral Sciences, Stanford University, Stanford, California

W. Stewart Agras, M.D.
Professor of Psychiatry (Emeritus), Department of Psychiatry and Behavioral Sciences, Stanford University, Stanford, California

Cara Bohon, Ph.D.
Assistant Professor, Department of Psychiatry and Behavioral Sciences, Stanford University, Stanford, California

Jennifer Derenne, M.D.
Clinical Associate Professor of Psychiatry and Behavioral Sciences, Stanford University School of Medicine, Stanford, California

Kathleen Kara Fitzpatrick, Ph.D.
Clinical Assistant Professor, Department of Psychiatry and Behavioral Sciences, Stanford University, Stanford, California

Nina Kirz, M.D.
Clinical Instructor, Eating Disorders Clinic, Department of Psychiatry and Behavioral Sciences, Stanford University School of Medicine, Stanford, California

James Lock, M.D., Ph.D.
Professor, Department of Psychiatry and Behavioral Sciences, Stanford University School of Medicine, Stanford, California

Lilya Osipov, Ph.D.
Clinical Instructor, Department of Psychiatry and Behavioral Sciences, Stanford University, Stanford, California

Athena Robinson, Ph.D.
Clinical Associate Professor, Eating Disorders Clinic, Department of Psychiatry and Behavioral Sciences, Stanford University School of Medicine, Stanford, California

Cristin D. Runfola, Ph.D.
Clinical Assistant Professor, Department of Psychiatry and Behavioral Sciences, Stanford University, Stanford, California

Debra L. Safer, M.D.
Associate Professor, Department of Psychiatry and Behavioral Sciences, Stanford University, Stanford, California

Hannah Welch
Assistant Clinical Research Coordinator, Department of Psychiatry and Behavioral Sciences, Stanford University, Stanford, California

Disclosure of Competing Interests

The following contributors to this book have indicated a financial interest in or other affiliation with a commercial supporter, a manufacturer of a commercial product, a provider of a commercial service, a nongovernmental organization, and/or a government agency, as listed below:

Sarah Adler, Psy.D.—*Royalties:* Guilford Press; *Research grant:* SPARK Spectrum study of binge-eating disorder (Qsymia)
Kathleen Kara Fitzpatrick, Ph.D.—Training Institute for Eating Disorders (payment for eating disorder training)
James Lock, M.D., Ph.D.—*Royalties:* Guilford Press, Oxford University Press, Routledge
Debra L. Safer, M.D.—*Royalties:* Guilford Press; *No salary support:* Spark Spectrum (repurposing Qsymia as treatment for BED)

The following contributors to this book have indicated that they have no financial interests or other affiliations that represent or could appear to represent a competing interest with their contributions to this book:

W. Stewart Agras, M.D.
Cara Bohon, Ph.D.
Jennifer Derenne, M.D.
Nina Kirz, M.D.
Lilya Osipov, Ph.D.
Athena Robinson, Ph.D.
Cristin D. Runfola, Ph.D.

Foreword

Providing care for any psychiatric disorder depends on accurate diagnosis and triage to the best available treatment. There is ample evidence that many psychiatric disorders, including the eating disorders, go unrecognized and thus untreated. As an illustration, a psychologist referred a young woman to me with a diagnosis of depression for a medication consultation. It turned out that the patient who had been receiving psychotherapy for over a year had a classic case of bulimia nervosa. When I asked why she hadn't talked about her eating disorder with her therapist, she replied, "My therapist never asked me about my eating, and I didn't want to talk about it." This vignette nicely illustrates one of the major problems in making an eating disorder diagnosis. If you don't ask about eating, then you may never hear about the patient's eating disorder. Even with all the publicity about eating disorders in the past several years, many will hide the disordered eating because of shame.

Diagnosis of a specific eating disorder is, of course, more complex, as is the further choice of an appropriate treatment and finding an adequate referral. This book offers a straightforward account of the diagnosis of the most common eating disorders with which patients and clients present to psychiatrists, psychologists, social workers, nutritionists, and physicians. The text provides a guide to the recognition of the eating disorders. In addition, consideration is given to short screening questionnaires and interview questions that are useful for detecting a problem with eating and alert the practitioner to follow-up with a more detailed history.

Although an eating disorder diagnosis may be made, access to treatment is often poor, and a number of studies have found that only a minority of individuals with eating disorders receive evidence-based care. As is the case in other prevalent psychiatric disorders, much of the triage and treatment of eating disorders will be in the hands of primary practitioners, including psychologists, internists, pediatricians, physicians and nutritionists. There are evidence-based treatments for all the eating disorders, and, with the exception of anorexia nervosa, effective briefer variants of treatment are available as described in this book. Although eating disorders are found across all ages, most eating disorders have their onset in adolescence or early adulthood. It seems likely that early identification and treatment will lead to better clinical outcomes. Again this book is written in the hope that the identification and treatment of individuals with eating disorders will improve.

The book is written in a format that allows quick access to basic information followed by a more detailed account of the topic. Chapters follow a standard format so that information for a particular eating disorder, such as the diagnostic features of a particular syndrome, medical and psychological comorbid entities, differential diagnosis, and evidence-based treatment, comes easily to hand. Reading a chapter introduction and reviewing the tables provides a quick guide to a particular disorder. Each of the major eating disorders are described in separate chapters, including anorexia nervosa, bulimia nervosa, binge-eating disorder, avoidant/restrictive food intake disorder, atypical eating disorders, and eating disorders in the context of obesity, again facilitating rapid access to the needed information.

For those interested in acquiring new skills to treat patients with eating disorders, resources for further training resources are provided at the end of each chapter.

W. Stewart Agras, M.D.

Preface

It may strike the reader as perhaps unusual to have the entire authorship of an edited book all from the same institution. Usually editors choose chapter authors from around the country or even the world to represent the very best knowledge and expertise in the field. In this case, however, that was not necessary—not because there are not remarkable experts in the eating disorder field around the country and the world, because there certainly are, and many of these excellent scientists and clinicians would have made outstanding contributions to this type of book. In this case, however, faculty members of Stanford's Department of Psychiatry and Behavioral Sciences who treat and conduct research related to eating disorders themselves represent such a rich repository of expertise in this field that it just was not necessary. The authors combined have more than 200 years of experience treating and conducting research in the field of eating disorders across the diagnostic and age spectrum. The median years of experience of the authors is 12 years of specialized clinical experience with eating disorders. In other words, as a clinician wanting an expert, experienced, and practical guide in the area of eating disorders, you are in good hands.

The level and depth of clinical and research experience is the product of a very long-standing commitment to the eating disorder population in Stanford's Department of Psychiatry and Behavioral Sciences. The earliest eating disorder treatment and research at Stanford dates back to 1972 with the arrival of Mickey Stunkard, M.D., and W. Stewart Agras, M.D., at Stanford (Adams et al. 1978; Agras et al. 1974). This gave rise to a stream of research in applications of behavior therapy to a variety of clinical problems and eventually to an eating disorders clinic and some of the first research into the treatment of bulimia nervosa with both medication and cognitive-behavioral therapy.

Treatment and research in the area of child and adolescent eating disorders stretch back to the founding of the eating disorder inpatient unit in 1978 by Hans Steiner, M.D., and Iris Litt, M.D. (Steiner et al. 1983). Over the course of 40 years, this program has been the training ground for child psychiatry, psychology, pediatric, and adolescent medicine clinicians (Lock and Steiner 1999). Ultimately, it also seeded the development of a large outpatient eating disorder clinic for youth that now comprises the lion's share of treatment for this age group in our department.

One of the key elements of the Stanford clinical and research activities in the area of eating disorders is the integration of these activities. The groundbreaking studies conducted here in bulimia nervosa (Agras and Dorian 1987; Agras et al. 2000; Le Grange et al. 2015), binge-eating disorders (Telch et al. 1990, 2000), and anorexia nervosa (Agras et al. 2014; Lock et al. 2005, 2010) were aimed most often at improving clinical practice and the care of patients with these disorders. The studies conducted aimed at clinical utility and relevance from the start. All the treatments described in the book were studied at Stanford (as well as other places of course) and specified through manuals that codified the therapeutic practices and processes (Agras and Apple 1997; Fitzpatrick et al. 2010; Le Grange and Lock 2007; Lock and Le Grange 2013; Safer et al. 2009). As a result, treatments described in this book are replicable and can be learned by studying these published manuals and by seeking further training and supervision.

Almost all the authors of this book served as treating clinicians and/or investigators on one or more of the pioneering studies of cognitive-behavioral therapy (CBT) or interpersonal psychotherapy for adults with bulimia nervosa, CBT or dialectical behavior therapy for adult binge-eating disorders, family-based treatment (FBT) or adolescent-focused treatment for anorexia nervosa or CBT, and/or FBT for adolescent bulimia nervosa. In other words, the authors are practicing clinicians and scientists who have made and continue to make contributions to the empirical evidence base guiding treatments for eating disorders.

Of course, the work—both clinical and research—aimed at improving our understanding of what causes and how best to evaluate and treat eating disorders goes on. Today we are exploring neurocognitive and neurobiological underpinnings of these disorders using expertise in cognitive neuroscience and neuroimaging (Garrett et al. 2013, 2014; Lock et al. 2011; Tchanturia and Lock 2011). We are also examining ways to improve current empirically supported treatments (Lock et al. 2013, 2015), widen access to effective treatments using technology (Darcy and Lock 2017; Lock et al. 2017), and develop novel treatments for conditions such as avoidant/

restrictive food intake disorder, or ARFID (Fitzpatrick et al. 2015). The authors of this book are involved in these myriad studies and will no doubt continue in the future to make important clinical and scientific contributions.

James Lock, M.D., Ph.D.

References

Adams N, Ferguson J, Stunkard AJ, Agras S: The eating behavior of obese and nonobese women. Behav Res Ther 16(4):225–232, 1978 718587

Agras WS, Apple RF: Overcoming Eating Disorders: A Cognitive-behavioral Treatment for Bulimia Nervosa and Binge Eating Disorder. Therapist Guide. San Antonio, TX., The Psychological Corporation, 1997

Agras WS, Dorian B: Imipramine in the treatment of bulimia: a double-blind controlled study. Int J Eat Disord 6:29–38, 1987

Agras WS, Barlow DH, Chapin HN, et al: Behavior modification of anorexia nervosa. Arch Gen Psychiatry 30(3):279–286, 1974 4813130

Agras WS, Walsh T, Fairburn CG, et al: A multicenter comparison of cognitive-behavioral therapy and interpersonal psychotherapy for bulimia nervosa. Arch Gen Psychiatry 57(5):459–466, 2000 10807486

Agras WS, Lock J, Brandt H, et al: Comparison of 2 family therapies for adolescent anorexia nervosa: a randomized parallel trial. JAMA Psychiatry 71(11):1279–1286, 2014 25250660

Darcy AM, Lock J: Using technology to improve treatment outcomes for children and adolescents with eating disorders. Child Adolesc Psychiatr Clin N Am 26(1):33–42, 2017 27837940

Fitzpatrick K, Moye A, Hoste R, et al: Adolescent focused therapy for adolescent anorexia nervosa. J Contemp Psychother 40:31–39, 2010

Fitzpatrick K, Forsberg S, Colborn D: Family-based treatment for Avoidant Restrictive Food Intake Disorder: families facing neophobias, in Family Therapy for Adolescent Eating and Weight Disorders: New Applications. Edited by Loeb K, Le Grange D, Lock J. New York, Routledge, 2015, pp 256–276

Garrett A, Datta N, Fitzpatrick K, et al: Brain activation associated with set-shifting and central coherence skills in patients with anorexia nervosa. Poster presented at the International Conference on Eating Disorders, Montreal, Canada, May 2013

Garrett AS, Lock J, Datta N, et al: Predicting clinical outcome using brain activation associated with set-shifting and central coherence skills in Anorexia Nervosa. J Psychiatr Res 57:26–33, 2014 25027478

Le Grange D, Lock J: Treating Bulimia in Adolescence. New York, Guilford, 2007

Le Grange D, Lock J, Agras WS, et al: Randomized clinical trial comparing family based treatment and cognitive behavioral therapy for adolescent bulimia nervosa. J Am Acad Child Adolesc Psychiatry 54(11):886.e2–894.e2, 2015 26506579

Lock J, Le Grange D: Treatment Manual for Anorexia Nervosa: A Family-Based Approach. New York, Guilford, 2013

Lock J, Steiner H (eds): Centre-Based Issue: Stanford University, Stanford, CA, USA: Clinical Child Psychology and Psychiatry. London, Sage, 1999

Lock J, Agras WS, Bryson S, Kraemer HC: A comparison of short- and long-term family therapy for adolescent anorexia nervosa. J Am Acad Child Adolesc Psychiatry 44(7):632–639, 2005 15968231

Lock J, Le Grange D, Agras WS, et al: Randomized clinical trial comparing family-based treatment with adolescent-focused individual therapy for adolescents with anorexia nervosa. Arch Gen Psychiatry 67(10):1025–1032, 2010 20921118

Lock J, Garrett A, Beenhakker J, Reiss AL: Aberrant brain activation during a response inhibition task in adolescent eating disorder subtypes. Am J Psychiatry 168(1):55–64, 2011 21123315

Lock J, Agras WS, Brandt H, et al: Addressing treatment dropout in anorexia nervosa using cognitive remediation therapy. Int J Eat Disord 46:567–575, 2013

Lock J, Le Grange D, Agras WS, et al: Can adaptive treatment imrove outcomes in family based treatment for adolescents with anorexia nervosa? Feasibility and treatment effects of a multi-site treatment study. Behav Res Ther 73:90–95, 2015

Lock J, Darcy A, Fitzpatrick KK, et al: Parental guided self-help family based treatment for adolescents with anorexia nervosa: A feasibility study. Int J Eat Disord 50(9):1104–1108, 2017 28580715

Safer DC, Telch F, Chen EY: Dialectical Behavior Therapy for Binge Eating and Bulimia. New York, Guilford, 2009

Steiner H, Walton CO, Emslie G: A psychosomatic unit for children and adolescents: report on first year and ten months. Child Psychiatry Hum Dev 14(1):3–15, 1983 6678710

Tchanturia K, Lock J: Cognitive remediation therapy for eating disorders: development, refinement and future directions. Curr Top Behav Neurosci 6:269–287, 2011 21243481

Telch CF, Agras WS, Rossiter EM, et al: Group cognitive-behavioral treatment for the nonpurging bulimic: an initial evaluation. J Consult Clin Psychol 58(5):629–635, 1990 2254511

Telch CF, Agras WS, Linehan MM: Group dialectical behavior therapy for binge eating disorder: a preliminary controlled trial. Behav Ther 31:569–582, 2000

How to Use This Book

Unfortunately, eating disorder evaluation and treatment is often sequestered in specialty clinics and programs despite the fact that these disorders are among the most common mental health problems, with a combined prevalence rate of approximately 10% (Smink et al. 2012). Most people with eating disorders do not have access to specialty services, and the majority of eating disorders go undiagnosed and untreated. Without treatment, eating disorders can lead to serious psychiatric, medical, and social disabilities (Campbell and Peebles 2014; Golden et al. 2003). Thus, it is important for clinicians who may not be specialists in eating disorders to develop an increased capacity to evaluate and treat these disorders as well as increase their understanding about what the needs of these patients are and refer to specialists when necessary. The hope is that this book will foster these increased capacities in practicing clinicians and further their interest in developing relevant clinical skills to help patients with eating disorders in their practices (von Ranson et al. 2013).

There are many books for specialist clinicians who treat persons with eating disorders. These are often wonderfully informative books, but because they are primarily aimed at a highly specialized professional audience, they can be impractical for clinicians who need to find the essentials more quickly. In addition, while the level of detail provided in these specialized texts is interesting to the expert, it can be an impediment for those who are not, making it difficult to see the forest for the trees. This book is squarely aimed at the big picture while highlighting the most important additional details.

This is a practical book to help the busy clinician quickly find the most relevant and up-to-date information about how to evaluate, diagnose, and treat people with eating disorders. The book will also be useful for those who regularly treat eating disorders but want a ready-to-hand reference and guide. Students in colleges, graduate programs, and postgraduate programs will also find this book an excellent primer on the presentation, epidemiology, risk factors, and major treatment approaches for eating disorders across the age spectrum.

The book is organized to make ease of access of information a major consideration. The first chapter provides an overview of all the major eating disorders and is a great place for the clinician to start his or her learning. It also includes a discussion of issues related to screening, race, culture, and gender that is cross-cutting and applicable to all the diagnostically themed chapters. Each of the remaining chapters focuses on a specific diagnostic group and is organized systematically to allow the reader to easily identify comparable elements across diagnostic groupings quickly. Thus, each chapter is structured with the following format:

Brief introduction: This short narrative section provides an overview of the main clinical features of each eating disorder grouping.

Key diagnostic checklist: This portion highlights the main diagnostic features of each diagnostic grouping.

Diagnostic rule outs: This portion identifies major diagnostic rule outs that should be considered in an evaluation/assessment process for each diagnostic grouping.

Epidemiology and risk factors: This portion provides bulleted information related to incidence, prevalence, and common risk factors for each diagnostic grouping.

Common comorbidities (medical and psychiatric): This portion lists the common medical and psychiatric problems that occur with each diagnostic grouping.

Clinical presentation(s): This section comprises short narrative clinical vignettes illustrating how patients within each diagnostic grouping typically present and includes variation of presentation by age specifically when warranted.

Evidence-based treatments: This portion summarizes the evidence-based interventions available for each diagnostic grouping and includes a ranking of the evidential base using the American Psychological Association criteria description of the level of evidence (Chambless and Ollendick 2001; Chorpita et al. 2011), as described further below.

Treatment settings and levels of care: This section summarizes the appropriate settings for initial treatment and required levels of care.

Treatments: This section describes the major evidence-based interventions for each diagnostic grouping.

Treatments illustrated: This section is composed of short narrative vignettes illustrating each of the major evidence-based interventions for each diagnostic grouping.

Clinical decision-making flowchart: Most chapters include a figure that illustrates the common decision tree for clinical management from presentation through discharge for each diagnostic grouping.

Common outcomes and complications: This portion lists common outcomes for each diagnostic grouping.

Resources and further reading: This section provides a list of resources for clinicians to access if additional information is needed related to each diagnostic grouping.

References: This section provides a list of references cited in the chapter.

With the exception of the first chapter, each chapter is designed to be self-contained. Thus, if you are interested in anorexia nervosa, the chapter on that diagnosis will contain all the pertinent information. This means in some cases there may be some overlap in content themes, but the application of content is specific to the chapter's diagnostic group. The diagnostic groups accorded a chapter are anorexia nervosa, bulimia nervosa, binge-eating disorder, and avoidant/restrictive food intake disorder. We also include special chapters on atypical eating disorders and eating disorders in the context of obesity.

Evidence-based treatments are emphasized in this book, and as mentioned earlier, evidential support is graded based on slightly modified criteria developed by the American Psychological Association (Chambless and Ollendick 2001; Chambless et al. 1996, 1998; Chorpita et al. 2011; Silverman and Hinshaw 2008). The main categories of evidence and their criteria are used in this book as follows:

Level 1: established treatment. Efficacy demonstrated by statistically superior findings in well-controlled randomized clinical trials or equivalent outcomes when compared with a well-established treatment.

Level 2: probably efficacious treatment. Two randomized controlled trials that demonstrate statistical superiority over wait-list control or one randomized controlled study showing statistical superiority over another active treatment.

Level 3: possibly efficacious treatment. One randomized controlled trial demonstrating statistical superiority over wait-list control or two clinical trials (nonrandomized) that show the treatment to be efficacious.

Level 4: experimental treatment. No randomized clinical trials and only one study showing the treatment to be efficacious in a nonrandomized study.

Level 5: questionable efficacy. Tested in randomized experiments and found to be inferior to other treatments or to wait list.

Each chapter author has used this grading scheme to rank the treatments they list and discuss. In most instances the evidence base for treatments is Level 2 or Level 3. In general, experimental treatments and treatments of questionable efficacy are not considered or discussed in detail. One area we have particularly emphasized is illustration of case presentations across the age spectrum, because many clinicians do not have the opportunity to see a full range of cases. A second area we highlight is treatment illustration. Again, how eating disorders are treated is often not well understood by many clinicians, so we have taken this opportunity to provide succinct case vignettes that illustrate how the most common and evidence-based interventions unfold.

We hope that in addition to being easy to use and practical, this book is enjoyable and helpful to all who use it.

James Lock, M.D., Ph.D.

References

Campbell K, Peebles R: Eating disorders in children and adolescents: state of the art review. Pediatrics 134(3):582–592, 2014 25157017

Chambless DL, Ollendick TH: Empirically supported psychological interventions: controversies and evidence. Annu Rev Psychol 52:685–716, 2001 11148322

Chambless DL, Sanderson W, Shoham V, et al: An update on empirically validated therapies. Clin Psychol 49:5–18, 1996

Chambless DL, Baker M, Baucom D, et al: Update on empirically validated therapies, II. Clin Psychol 51(1):3–16, 1998

Chorpita B, Daleiden E, Ebesutani C, et al: Evidence-based treatments for children and adolescents: an updated review of indicators of efficacy and effectiveness. Clin Psychol Sci Pract 18(2):154–172, 2011

Golden NH, Katzman DK, Kreipe RE, et al: Eating disorders in adolescents: position paper of the Society for Adolescent Medicine. J Adolesc Health 33(6):496–503, 2003 14642712

Silverman W, Hinshaw S: The second special issue on evidence-based psychosocial treatments for children and adolescents: a 10-year update. J Clin Child Adolesc Psychol 37(1):1–7, 2008

Smink FR, van Hoeken D, Hoek HW: Epidemiology of eating disorders: incidence, prevalence and mortality rates. Curr Psychiatry Rep 14(4):406–414, 2012 22644309

von Ranson KM, Wallace LM, Stevenson A: Psychotherapies provided for eating disorders by community clinicians: infrequent use of evidence-based treatment. Psychother Res 23(3):333–343, 2013 23088433

Chapter 1

Eating Disorders

The Basics

James Lock, M.D., Ph.D.
Lilya Osipov, Ph.D.

Introduction

This chapter provides both an overall introduction to all eating disorders and a single reference point for any reader seeking a quick overview of the clinical presentations, diagnostic criteria, major treatment options, treatment prognosis, and general resources for eating disorders. As in every chapter, all major points are presented in brief tabular form in highlighted portions of the text for easy referencing. We begin with a very brief timeline of the diagnostic evolution of eating disorders. The timeline is followed by a summary of the presenting features of each of the major disorders and the best treatment approach based on the current evidence base.

Richard Morton, in a case series published in 1689, described the clinical manifestations of young patients suffering from behaviors and cognitions he called "nervous consumption" (Morton 1694), which are consistent with what we now recognize as anorexia nervosa (AN). However, the term *anorexia nervosa* itself was coined by Sir William Gull in England in 1874, with the term *anorexia hysterique* introduced by Charles Lesegue in France at nearly the same time (Gull 1874). *Bulimia nervosa* (BN) was first included in DSM-III in 1980 (American Psychiatric Association 1980) following clinical descriptions of patients with binge eating and purging by Boskind-Lodahl ("bulimarexia") (Boskind-Lodahl 1976; Boskind-Lodahl and White 1978) and Russell, who called it "an ominous variant" of AN (Russell 1979). Binge-eating disorder (BED) was systematically described in 1959 by Albert Stunkard (1959), who characterized it as a pattern of abnormal eating found in patients with obesity. BED was not included in DSM, however, until the fourth edition (DSM-IV, American Psychiatric Association 1994). At that point it was introduced as a provisional diagnosis requiring further study within the category "Eating Disorder Not Otherwise Specified" (EDNOS). BED was officially added as a distinct, stand-alone diagnosis in DSM-5 (American Psychiatric Association 2013). The most recent addition to the diagnostic classification of eating problems is avoidant/restrictive food intake disorder (ARFID), which was added to DSM-5 in 2013. This is an eating disorder found principally in children. In ARFID, food or eating is avoided, usually leading to low weight, but the avoidance is not associated with shape or weight concerns or intentional efforts to reduce weight (Bryant-Waugh and Kreipe 2012).

Screening

Screening of patients for eating disorders in the context of evaluations is important. Eating disorders are commonly hidden from others and sometimes felt to shameful. As a result, many eating disorders are undetected even by professionals treating patients with these disorders for related conditions such as depression, anxiety, and trauma. Therefore, it is important that mental health practitioners include screening questions about eating disorders in their general assessments. Simple questions such as those on the Eating Disorder Screen for Primary Care (ESP; Cotton et al. 2003) can be readily incorporated into a baseline clinical interview (e.g., Are you satisfied with your eating pattern? Do you ever eat in secret? Does your weight affect the way you feel about yourself? Have any members of your family had an eating disorder? Do you currently have or have you had an eating disorder?). There are also short questionnaires that can be used as paper-and-pen or online approaches when assessing new patients. One of these is the SCOFF, which consists of five short questions and has demonstrated good reliability (Morgan et al. 1999). The Eating Disorder Examination—Questionnaire (EDE-Q), Eating Disorder Inventory (EDI), and Eating Attitudes Test (EAT) are validated, short, self-report measures that can be useful screening instruments for eating disorders (Garner et al. 1982, 1983; Passi et al. 2003). Because many eating disorders begin during preteen and adolescent years, screening this high-at-risk group is critical. The Kids' Eating Disorders Survey (KEDS) and the children's version of the EDE-Q (ChEDE-Q), EDI (EDI-C), and the EAT (ChEAT) are all validated measures for use in younger children (Childress et al. 1993). It is also wise to ask parents if they have concerns about their children's eating or weight as a screening strategy.

Major Eating and Feeding Disorders

Anorexia Nervosa

AN is the least common of the eating disorders, but it is the most lethal (Smink et al. 2012) It typically has its onset in the late childhood and early adolescent years, and it is rare for new cases to arise after the age of 25 years (van Son et al. 2006). Nonetheless, with a prevalence of approximately 1% in adolescent females, AN is almost as common as schizophrenia. It is reported in all parts of the world at similar incidence rates, although some data suggest that persons of African descent may be less vulnerable (Hoek et al. 2005).

AN is one of the oldest of the psychiatric diagnoses, having been first described in the medical literature almost 150 years ago (Gull 1874). Interestingly, although some of the specific criteria for diagnosing AN have changed over time, the main features of the disorder are fundamentally unchanged. There appears to a relatively strong genetic component contributing to the risk for the disorder (Trace et al. 2013). Similarly, there appear to be few cultural variations in the expression of the disorder, although changes in expression over long stretches of time may be present. In this regard, "holy anorexia"—that is, self-starvation as a form of self-mortification to worship Christ—was observed in the Middle Ages (Saraf 1998). In this context, the behaviors associated with self-starvation were associated with cognitions related to worship as opposed to appearance. Nonetheless, the persistence of these behaviors and the necessary ability to deny oneself food to the point of severe malnutrition are shared across time. In this sense, starvation itself likely reinforces food, eating, and weight preoccupation, as reports of the starved conscientious objectors in Ancel Keys' experiment demonstrated (Keys et al. 1950)

The key features of the disorder are a determined effort to radically diminish the ratio of energy intake and increase energy output so that a negative balance leads to clinically significant weight loss. Behaviors include undergoing severe dieting, eating only foods with low caloric density, decreasing portion sizes, increasing exercise, and purging by vomiting, laxative use, or exercise (American Psychiatric Association 2013). In younger children and adolescents, weight loss may not be great but still lead to medical compromise, growth delay, and other psychological and social problems (Nicholls et al. 2000). In adults and most adolescents, once AN has been established, it is accompanied by fear and anxiety about eating that can be behaviorally and emotionally severely disorganizing. These behaviors are associated with a preoccupation with weight and sometimes shape. Many times, however, these preoccupations are related to *internal* rather than external standards. For example, a person with AN may want to lose weight as a personal achievement, ever aiming to reach a lower weight (Halmi et al. 2012) regardless of the effect on her appearance. This distinguishes the motivations of persons with AN from those of persons with other eating disorders such as BN, which are often driven by wishes to be attractive in the eyes of others. Typically, those who develop AN have a history of academic and/or athletic accomplishment with strong internal drives for achievement in terms of grades and other types of socially sanctioned rewards. AN is described as an ego-syntonic disorder—a disorder characterized by a refusal to acknowledge the problems associated with AN and an unwillingness to engage in treatment. These features make treatment of AN particularly challenging.

Despite the long history of identifying AN as a severe psychiatric problem, studies of treatments are few (Watson and Bulik 2013). For the first 100 years since AN was described by Gull, treatment mostly consisted of very long (i.e., many years in duration) hospitalization (McKenzie and Joyce 1992). Families were seen as likely etiological agents or as ineffective and barriers to treatment. Psychoanalytic approaches were in vogue for a period but not particularly effective (Bruch 1973; Thoma 1967). Many medications have been tried, particularly those with side effects of weight gain, in the hope that this would help patients recover, but data have yet to identify any medication with systematic benefits (Hay and Claudino 2012). Cognitive-behavioral therapy (CBT) is a mainstay treatment for other eating disorders, but its effects for AN appear more limited, probably in part because CBT requires commitment and motivation for recovery on the part of patients, which is often severely lacking in those with AN (Fairburn et al. 2002). It also appears that longer duration of AN leads to decreasing responsiveness to treatment as the person with AN becomes more and more identified with the disorder over the developmental period from adolescence through adulthood (Hay 2013).

There is greater hope for successful treatment of AN when it is treated early and effectively (Treasure and Russell 2011). The approach that has demonstrated the most success to date with young adolescents with AN with a short course of treatment is family-based treatment (FBT) (Lock 2015; Lock and Le Grange 2013). This treatment overcomes the lack of motivation on the patient's part by helping parents refeed the patient at home, much as nurses would have done in a hospital. However, the difference between refeeding at home and in the hospital is crucial, because it is clear that learning to eat in a hospital setting, while potentially lifesaving, does not typically generalize to eating at home. This lack of generalizability has been well demonstrated, as the long history of weight loss after weight restoration in hospital has amply demonstrated. Other approaches, such as adolescent-focused therapy (AFT; Fitzpatrick et al. 2009; Lock et al. 2010) and systemic family therapy (SyFT; Pote et al. 2001), are also effective, although they are slower and appear to be more expensive to provide (Agras et al. 2014).

If AN is treated early, the prognosis is reasonably good, with full recovery rates in the range of 40%–50% and another 30%–35% substantially improved. On the other hand, once the illness becomes protracted, treatment response is more limited (Hay et al. 2012) and is associated with severe psychological, social, and medical problems, including the highest mortality rate of the psychiatric diagnoses (Arcelus et al. 2011).

Bulimia Nervosa

Although bulimic behaviors have been documented since ancient times (Russell 1997), the diagnosis of BN was proposed only in the 1970s (Russell 1979). Nevertheless, BN is more common than AN, with a reported incidence rate of about 1% and a prevalence rate of about 3% (Hoek and van Hoeken 2003). Like AN, the disorder is more prevalent in young women, but males make up between 10% and 30% of individuals with the disorder. Bulimic behaviors typically have their onset at about age 16 years (Stice and Agras 1998).

BN is characterized by recurrent episodes of overeating in a discrete period of time accompanied by a feeling of being unable to control eating (American Psychiatric Association 2013).

Following these overeating episodes, purgative behaviors, including vomiting, laxative use, and exercise, are used to try to compensate for the caloric intake associated with a binge-eating episode. These behaviors are usually accompanied by feelings of guilt and shame. Unlike AN, the disorder is almost always ego-dystonic—that is, the patient recognizes these behaviors as problematic and wishes to change them. Patients with BN are dissatisfied by their weight and appearance and wish to change it to be more attractive. These overvaluations of weight and of shape are key elements in self-worth and core elements in the diagnosis of BN.

Bulimic behaviors become increasingly habitual over time and are often used to manage emotional states such as anger, frustration, and loss. Generalizing bulimic behaviors as a coping strategy to manage these other emotional states increases their value and makes them more challenging to change. In addition, BN is associated with high degrees of psychiatric comorbidity, particularly depression and anxiety disorders. Impulse-control disorder problems and substance abuse are also common (Le Grange and Lock 2002).

Although BN was described as a distinct clinical syndrome almost 100 years later than AN, progress on treatment is considerably more advanced for BN than for AN (Hay et al. 2009). In part, this is a result of the fortuitous timing of the evolution of CBT with the identification of BN. CBT in various formats has been shown to be effective for both adolescents and adults with BN. CBT initially focuses on maintaining behaviors through providing psychoeducation, self-monitoring food intake, and establishing a regular pattern of eating. Next, CBT aims to address maintaining distorted beliefs and thoughts about the impact of eating, appearance, and weight on personal, social, and interpersonal interactions and self-worth. In general, about 30%–35% of persons with BN fully recover when treated with CBT. Other treatments are also effective, including interpersonal psychotherapy (IPT), but treatment response is slower (Agras et al. 2000). Antidepressants are also useful for BN, but they are not as effective as CBT (Hay and Claudino 2012). Thus, most guidelines recommend antidepressants as an adjunctive treatment to psychological interventions. For adolescents, FBT that is modified for BN is more effective than CBT, at least in the short term (Le Grange et al. 2015). In FBT for BN, adjustments to the approach are made to account for the older age of most of the patients, which is associated with greater age-appropriate autonomy; the ego-dystonic nature of the disorder, which allows for more active participation of the adolescent in behavioral management; as well as the need to take a broader clinical focus than in AN to address symptoms of depression and anxiety that are commonly present (Le Grange and Lock 2007).

Although many individuals recover from BN, there is a moderate chance of recurrent episodes after even long periods of recovery. Periods of stress and emotional upheaval or loss, as well as changes in life circumstances such as moving or starting college, are associated with increased risk of both onset and relapse of BN (Halmi et al. 2002).

Binge-Eating Disorder

BED was added to DSM as a research diagnosis or provisional diagnosis in DSM-IV, published in 1994, even though it had been recognized as early as 1959 as a behavior associated with obesity (Stunkard 1959). BED was recognized as an eating disorder distinct from BN because although binge-eating behavior is common to both, BED lacks compensatory behaviors (e.g., vomiting, laxative use, over-exercise). Also, BN requires that the patient report overvaluation of self-worth based on weight and shape, and this is not a requirement for BED.

Binge eating is defined as eating an objectively large amount of food accompanied by a feeling of loss of control over eating—a sense that one cannot stop eating—over a discrete period of time (e.g., 1–2 hours). These episodes are not culturally sanctioned overeating (e.g., feasting for holidays) and must occur at least one time per week over a period of 3 months or more. In addition, binge eating is accompanied by at least three of the following: rapid eating, eating to the point of physical discomfort, eating without hunger, eating alone to avoid embarrassment about food consumption, and feelings of depression, disgust, and guilt after a binge-eating episode. These episodes must also lead to significant emotional distress, physical, or social impairment.

BED is among the most common of the eating disorders, with a lifetime prevalence of about 3% (Swanson et al. 2011). BED has the latest age at onset of the eating disorders, at about 23 years, despite the fact that binge-eating episodes commonly start in the middle teenage years (Stice and Agras 1998). BED is multifactorial in terms of etiology, with heritable, familial, and social contributors for risk. Psychiatric comorbidity is also common, with depression, anxiety, and substance abuse disorders among the most common (Telch and Stice 1998). Medical problems associated with obesity appear to worsen with BED and include hypertension, diabetes, sleep disorders, and joint problems.

BED is a highly treatable condition, although treatments appear to be effective for binge-eating behavior rather than associated obesity (Vocks et al. 2010). CBT (Agras and Apple 1997), IPT (Wilfley et al. 2002), and dialectical behavior therapy (DBT) (Safer et al. 2009) are all helpful. Both CBT and IPT follow the same general principles as in BN described earlier. DBT addresses binge eating as a maladaptive strategy for managing unpleasant emotional states and aims to help patients develop skills to better manage distressful emotional states (Safer et al. 2007). Interventions include teaching mindfulness, distress tolerance, emotion regulation, and interpersonal effectiveness. Data supporting the use of DBT are more limited than those for CBT or IPT but are growing (Safer et al. 2010; Telch et al. 2000, 2001), with promising binge-eating abstinence rates found posttreatment (Grilo 2017).

Pharmacological treatments are also commonly used in BED. Only lisdexamfetamine dimesylate (LDX), a stimulant originally indicated for attention-deficit/hyperactivity disorder (ADHD), is currently approved by the U.S. Food and Drug Administration (FDA) for treating BED, and only in adults. Antidepressants, anticonvulsants, and antiobesity agents have also demonstrated efficacy in randomized clinical trials and are now used as off-label treatments. A comprehensive review of these studies has recently been published by McElroy (2017).

The prognosis of BED is variable. Many if not most patients with BED are never diagnosed or receive treatment. Unfortunately, medical complications and related expenses are common (Ágh et al. 2016; Ling et al. 2017). Younger patients with BED are at greater risk for obesity, depression, and substance use and abuse (Sonneville et al. 2012).

Avoidant/Restrictive Food Intake Disorder

ARFID is a new diagnosis in DSM-5 (see Bryant-Waugh and Kreipe 2012; Bryant-Waugh et al. 2010; Kreipe and Palomaki 2012). The distinguishing diagnostic feature of ARFID from other eating disorders is food restriction or avoidance without accompanying shape or weight concerns or intentional efforts to lose weight. Nonetheless, ARFID is associated with significant weight loss and nutritional deficiencies as well as emotional and psychological dysfunction. There are three main presentations of ARFID: highly selective or picky eating; extreme fear of choking or swallowing; and/or extreme undereating due to low appetite. Some patients with ARFID report neophobia related to novel food types or are hypersensitive to food texture, appearance, and taste (Bryant-Waugh and Nicholls 2011; Faith 2010; Kreipe and Palomaki 2012; Nicholls et al. 2001). ARFID patients who present with a swallowing or choking phobia have usually experienced a medical procedure that caused choking, an allergic reaction that led to throat closure, or a severe gagging after trying to swallow. Fear that food will cause this frightening event to recur leads to avoidance of eating. Individuals who show little interest in food or experience little appetite can also be diagnosed with ARFID. Often these are lifelong eating patterns that have been accepted as normal despite the negative health impacts.

Each of these presentations of ARFID have unique clinical challenges, and there are no empirical studies available to date to guide treatment. At this time, treatment is highly individualized and designed to address specific behavioral and emotional reactions that are interfering with adequate nutritional intake. A few clinical reports suggest that CBT, exposure/prevention behavioral plans, and FBT might be useful (Nicholls et al. 2001).

Key Diagnostic Checklist

Anorexia nervosa

❏ Inadequate nutrition intake relative to energy needs.

❏ Significantly low weight or failure to attain expected growth.

❏ Intense fear of weight gain or becoming overweight, or behavior that interferes with weight gain.

❏ Disturbance in perception of weight or shape, undue influence of weight and shape on self-evaluation, or inability to recognize the severity of low weight.

- *Restricting subtype*—weight loss achieved through restriction and/or excessive exercise.

- *Binge-eating/purging subtype*—engagement in recurrent binge-eating or purging (inducing vomiting or use of laxatives, diuretics, emetics) over preceding 3 months.

Bulimia nervosa

❏ Recurrent episodes of both binge eating and inappropriate compensatory behaviors. Binge episodes are time limited and are associated with a loss of control over eating. Compensatory behaviors (e.g., vomiting, laxatives, excessive exercise) are undertaken to compensate for overeating. These behaviors occur at least once per week over the course of 3 months.

❏ Concerns about body shape and weight that contribute highly to self-evaluation.

Binge-eating disorder

Binge eating (large amount of food + loss of control) occurring at least once per week for a minimum of 3 months in the absence of compensatory behaviors (American Psychiatric Association 2015). In children and adolescents, loss of control over eating appears a better clinical marker of binge eating than amount of food consumed (Marcus and Kalarchian 2003).

❏ Association of BED with at least three of five other features, including eating much more quickly than normal, eating until the point of physical discomfort, eating despite lack of physical hunger, eating alone due to embarrassment about one's amount of food intake, and feeling disgust, depression, or guilt after binge eating.

❏ Distress and/or impairment in functioning due to binge-eating symptoms.

Avoidant/restrictive food intake disorder

❏ Disturbance in perception of weight or shape, undue influence of weight and shape on self-evaluation, or inability to recognize the severity of low weight.

❏ Significant, ongoing, difficulty with feeding/eating behaviors that results in one of the following:

• Failure to make appropriate weight gain or significant weight loss.

• Inability to meet nutritional needs, resulting in nutritional deficiency.

• Ability to meet nutritional or energy needs only with use of oral nutritional supplements or enteral feeds.

- Feeding/eating behaviors that result in significant impairment in psychosocial functioning.

❏ No body image disturbance.

❏ No current anorexia nervosa/bulimia nervosa.

❏ Not due to a medical illness, cultural practice, or lack of available nutrition.

Psychiatric Rule Outs

- Major depressive disorder
- Psychotic disorders
- Substance use disorders
- Anxiety disorders (e.g., generalized anxiety, social anxiety disorder)
- Obsessive-compulsive and related disorders (e.g., obsessive compulsive disorder, body dysmorphic disorder)

Epidemiology and Risk Factors

Epidemiology

- Anorexia nervosa
  - AN has a prevalence of 0.5%–1.5% in young women (Smink et al. 2014). Current estimates suggest that the ratio of females to males is 10:1 (Hatmaker 2005; Lock 2008).
- Bulimia nervosa
  - BN has a 12-month prevalence of 1%–1.5% among adolescent and young adult women (American Psychiatric Association 2013). Lifetime bulimia nervosa prevalence rates in the National Comorbidity Survey—Replication were 0.5% and 1.3% among boys and girls, respectively (Swanson et al. 2011).
- Binge-eating disorder
  - Binge-eating disorder is the most common of the eating disorders. Among adults in the United States, life-

time prevalence estimates range from 1.52% to 2.6% and 12-month prevalence estimates range from 1.2% to 1.64% depending on study and diagnostic criteria (i.e., DSM-IV vs. DSM-5). In adolescents, the lifetime prevalence is 2.3% in females and 0.8% in males (Swanson et al. 2011).

- Avoidant/restrictive food intake disorder
  - There are as of this writing no epidemiological data available for ARFID.

Risk Factors

- *Biological factors:* Genetic vulnerability in first-degree relatives of those with an eating disorder; weight loss may also precipitate disordered eating; hormonal changes associated with puberty and later life may also confer some risk.
- *Psychological factors:* Perfectionistic, harm-avoidant, and self-doubting temperaments increase risk (Anderluh et al. 2003); separations and transitions, as well as stressful life events such as moving, taking on a new job, or dealing with the loss of a loved one, may increase risk as well.
- *Social and environmental factors:* Societal preoccupation with thinness; dieting (Jones et al. 2004); or participation in activities that involve a desired body type or weight class (such as wrestling, rowing, gymnastics, figure skating, or ballet) increases risk.

Common Comorbidities

Medical

- Malnutrition
- Electrolyte abnormalities
- Hypo- or hypertension
- Orthostasis
- Obesity
- Bradycardia, prolonged QTc, dysrhythmia
- Osteoporosis

- Refeeding syndrome—phosphate and magnesium may decrease because of shifts related to renourishment
- Vitamin D deficiency

Psychiatric

- Mood disorders (particularly depression and bipolar disorder)—care must be taken to screen and monitor for suicidal ideation, as many patients with eating disorders die by suicide.
- Anxiety disorders
- Obsessive-compulsive disorder
- Substance use disorders
- Personality disorders

Evidence-Based Outpatient Treatments for Eating Disorders

Anorexia Nervosa

Cognitive-behavioral therapy for adults (Fairburn et al. 2008)—Level 3 (possibly efficacious)

Focal psychodynamic individual therapy for adults (Zipfel et al. 2014)—Level 3 (possibly efficacious)

Family-based treatment for adolescents (Lock and Le Grange 2013)—Level 1 (established treatment)

Adolescent-focused treatment for adolescents (Fitzpatrick et al. 2009)—Level 3 (possibly efficacious)

Systemic family therapy for adolescents (Agras et al. 2014)—Level 3 (possibly efficacious)

Cognitive-behavioral therapy for adolescents (Gowers et al. 2007)—Level 3 (possibly efficacious)

Bulimia Nervosa

Cognitive-behavioral therapy for adults (Fairburn et al. 2008)—Level 1 (established treatment)

Interpersonal psychotherapy for adults (Agras et al. 2000)—Level 1 (established treatment)

Dialectical behavior therapy for adults (Safer et al. 2001)—Level 3 (possibly efficacious)

Family-based treatment for adolescents (Le Grange et al. 2015)—Level 3 (possibly efficacious)

Cognitive-behavioral therapy for adolescents (Fairburn et al. 2008)—Level, 3 (possibly efficacious)

Antidepressants—Level 1, established treatment (in adults); Level 4 (experimental treatment [in adolescents])

Binge-Eating Disorder

Cognitive-behavioral therapy (Fairburn et al. 2008)—established treatment

Interpersonal psychotherapy (Rieger et al. 2010)—probably efficacious

Dialectical behavior therapy (Safer et al. 2009)—probably efficacious

Behavioral weight loss (Peat et al. 2017)—probably efficacious

Psychopharmacological therapy—Level 1 (established treatment)

Avoidant/Restrictive Food Intake Disorder

Family-based treatment (Fitzpatrick et al. 2015)—Level 4 (experimental treatment)

Cognitive-behavioral therapy (Thomas et al. 2017)—Level 4 (experimental treatment)

Eating Disorders in Ethnic and Cultural Minorities, Males, and Sexual and Gender Minorities

Eating disorders affect individuals of all ages, races, sexual orientations, and gender presentations. Our aim in this section is to help clinicians consider sociocultural factors when they are working with individuals with eating disorders. Our overall recommendation is that clinicians strive to provide culturally sensitive treatments, refer to source materials, and also consider their patient's experience, self-conceptualization, and identity. To date, treatments for eating disorders have been developed and studied in largely white, middle-class, heterosexual populations (Reyes-Rodríguez et al. 2010). A goal of this chapter is to enhance case formulation for treatment by helping clinicians to be cognizant of how different concerns, such as sexual orientation, socioeconomic status, and cultural beliefs, may affect symptoms presentation, patient perspectives, and engagement in treatment as well as to have an increased appreciation for how the patient's social supports (family, culture, ethnic identity) may impact treatment.

Ethnic and Cultural Minorities

Eating disorders and maladaptive eating behaviors are found in all ethnic and racial groups. Degree of acculturation, stress related to immersion in a new culture, cultural identification, and other sociocultural variables may impact symptoms presentation, identification, and willingness to seek treatment as well as engagement and response to different therapeutic modalities (Franko et al. 2007; Perez and Plasencia 2016). Individuals from non-Western backgrounds may struggle to reconcile their culture of origin's body image ideals with other, frequently slimmer, body image ideals that are presented in the media and are endorsed by peers and others in Western culture and to which there is perceived pressure to conform. The distress experienced by individuals is moderated by other variables, including family structure and immersion in the family system, body composition, and meaning assigned to food and eating (Soh et al. 2006).

Recent data suggest that some ethnic minority groups are particularly vulnerable to developing eating disorders and disordered eating behaviors. In the United States, prevalence rates of eating disorders and associated features (body dissatisfaction, drive for thinness, weight shape concerns) in Latina women appear similar to those of other white women (Gordon et al. 2010; Perez et al. 2016), with BED being the most common eating disorder diagnosed in this group—1.92% for lifetime prevalence of BED and 5.61% for prevalence of any binge-eating behavior (Alegria et al. 2007). Some Latinas may struggle to reconcile the curve and slender figure they perceive as the Latin cultural ideal with the ideal attributed to the American culture—that is, the thin beauty ideal (Gordon et al. 2010). Moreover, in Latino culture there is often a strong connection between family members/generations, with food preparation and eating communicating love, care, and belonging to a larger group, and this could lead to fears of social isolation or rejection if an eating disorder develops (Reyes-Rodríguez et al. 2016).

To date, findings suggest that African American women are buffered somewhat from the development of AN, with low lifetime prevalence of AN in this group (0.17%) relative to their white counterparts (Taylor et al. 2007). As among Latinas, BED is the most common eating disorder reported in this ethnic/racial group (Striegel-Moore et al. 2003). Lifetime estimates for BED are 1.66% for BED and 5.08% for any binge eating (Taylor et al. 2007). Some studies suggest that rates of BN among African Americans women are comparable to those of white women, but findings are inconclusive. When eating disorders are present in African Americans, symptom profiles mostly appear to be similar to those observed in white women. This may be particularly true for AN and may reflect the strong physiological and genetic component implicated in the etiology of this disorder. African American women with BN appear to have shorter illness duration, higher rates of sexual abuse history, lower frequency of comorbid substance use, higher body mass index (BMI), and higher rates of depression relative to white individuals with BN (Chui et al. 2007; Dohm et al. 2002; Hudson et al. 2007). With respect to BED, black and African women with BED present with similar comorbidities and impairments across domains of functioning as white individuals. Relative to their white counterparts, African American women report significantly higher stress, more critical comments about weight and eating from others, and greater prevalence of pregnancy in the 12 months prior to binge-eating onset (Pike et al. 2006). As a result of these findings, it has been suggested that binge eating in African Americans may sometimes represent a maladaptive coping response to life stressors rather than a behavior driven by weight/shape concerns. In African American women, BED is also associated with shorter duration of illness, later age at onset, higher BMI, fewer and less severe depressive symptoms, and higher self-esteem (Franko et al. 2012).

Even less is known about epidemiology of eating disorders among Asian Americans. Available data appear to challenge the notion that Asian American women display a lower prevalence of eating-related concerns or present with less severe clinical profiles. Marques et al. (2011) reported that lifetime prevalence of eating disorders in Asian Americans is similar to that observed in white samples, with lifetime prevalence rates of 0.10% for AN, 1.50% for BN, and 1.24% for BED in the former. Studies are inconclusive about the levels of body dissatisfaction and disordered eating in this ethnic group (Akan and Grilo 1995; Grabe and Hyde 2006). As with other cultural groups, it is essential to consider the meaning assigned to eating as well as culture-specific values and norms. It has been suggested that in some instances, eating disorders symptoms in Asians and Asian American (and others disorders involving somatic symptoms) may be culturally sanctioned ways of expressing other emotions, such as depression and anxiety (see Yokoyama 2007). Among Asian American women presenting for treatment, the focus sometimes appears to be on specific body parts rather than overall shape or weight (Mintz and Kashubeck 1999).

A recent systematic review by Sinha and Warfa (2013) of 12 qualitative and quantitative studies of treatment utilization among ethnic minority individuals concluded that members of ethnic minority groups are less likely to seek and receive treatment as well as less likely to be referred to services specific to eating disorders than their white counterparts. Among immigrant populations and ethnic minority individuals, acculturation immigration status, understanding of eating disorders, stigma, lack of health insurance or access to healthcare, as well as underutilization of health services in general, are barriers to timely diagnosis and treatment (Reyes-Rodríguez et al. 2013). For example, Cachelin et al. (2000) reported that more acculturated women are both significantly more likely to suffer from any eating disorder and more likely to seek and receive treatment compared with less acculturated women.

Patients from these more diverse backgrounds may first attempt to seek the advice of trusted others regardless of their level of knowledge and expertise. Patients may also be caught in a bind between trying to follow culturally endorsed norms of eating to abundance, celebrating with food, striving for curvier body image ideal, and responding to their perceptions of what is expected in the mainstream Western culture (George and Franko 2010). This tension may increase feelings of guilt and shame and impede individuals from seeking help for their eating disorder. With respect to detection and assessment of eating disorders and related symptoms, rates of diagnoses are limited by the diagnostic criteria that reflect eating disorder features salient in the Western cultures. In addition, assessment measures that were developed to assess eating disorders in white samples are often not validated for us with other ethnic or cultural or racial groups. One example of this is that among Asians, some studies suggest that an intense fear of fatness may be less relevant to assessing eating disorders (Lee 1995).

There are limited data regarding the efficacy of extant empirically validated treatments in nonwhite populations. Moreover, translating evidence-based treatments to real-world settings is further hindered by previously mentioned challenges, including access to services, economic barriers to treatment attendance and engagement, cultural beliefs that promote stigma and shame in the patient, or the sociocultural milieu. Currently, adopting and applying evidence-supported interventions with members of ethnic minority groups is generally appropriate, while keeping in mind cultural values and patient's/family's adherence to these values, acculturation, experiences related to discrimination, and potential barriers to treatment. In general, the clinician may benefit from consulting the American Psychological Association (2017) guidelines on multiculturalism.

Data support the efficacy of FBT for adolescent AN and BN (Lock 2010; Lock and Le Grange 2005). Although there are no randomized, controlled studies looking at efficacy of family-based interventions for members of ethnic minority groups, data do not suggest that race or ethnicity moderates treatment outcomes. Secondary analyses of efficacy data by Doyle et al. (2009) found that FBT yielded reduction in eating disorder behaviors and depressive symptoms in African American youth with BN. Individuals and families from cultures in which the family plays a central role, such as the Latino culture, may respond particularly well to the principles of FBT. Traditional values in the Latino culture promote children's dependence on parents, including in the realm of eating and treatment adherence (Reyes-Rodríguez and Bulik 2010). On the other hand, in both the Latino and Asian American cultures, there may be a tendency to defer to the clinician as the "expert" who will address the problem by telling the young patient to eat. Indeed, clinical experience suggests that less acculturated families may at times become frustrated with FBT's focus on a) externalizing the illness by shifting blame away from the patient, and b) the clinician's adopting a consultant stance aimed at empowering parents to renourish their child rather than providing specific instructions and guidelines for "what to do." Because perception of acceptance may be particularly important for Latino patients, the clinician should encourage warmth and acceptance of the patient within the family regardless of the patient's eating challenges.

There is also a scarcity of providers fluent in languages other than English. Although many second-generation patients and children are fluent in English, many parents are non-English speaking. Thus, the clinician is faced with the challenge of working with an interpreter, relying on a third party to deliver the information in the intended manner and tone. Many ethnic minority individuals may also face socioeconomic challenges that may affect their ability to attend sessions on a regular basis, provide the quantities of food necessary to facilitate weight progress, and travel to appointments. Others may have more limited education and knowledge about nutrition and thus can be more easily led astray by the child with the eating disorder, particularly if meal planning recommendations are not based on foods endemic to the culture. As part of treatment it is important to assess parents' understanding of their child's illness and barriers to making weight progress and families' expectations of different members of the treatment team. In some immigrant families, the patient is an older adolescent who is taking care of younger siblings while one or both parents are working, and thus a parent is not available to supervise meals. Because family is often so central in the Latino culture, it is important to explore with parents if members of extended family are available to provide support and supervision.

With respect to other evidence-supported treatment modalities, recently there has been an effort to adapt CBT for BN for Hispanic and Latino patients (Shea et al. 2012). The authors' recommendations for adapting CBT are congruent with clinical observations in delivering FBT with Latino and Hispanic families and include a) increasing family and peer involvement, b) adapting meal plans to reflect culturally preferred foods that are readily available and affordable, and c) addressing issues pertinent to acculturative stress and cultural differences in body image ideals (Perez and Plasencia 2016).

One randomized controlled study compared CBT and IPT for the treatment of BN for African American individuals. Chui et al. (2007) reported that relative to IPT, CBT was associated with higher rates of abstinence from binge eating and purging in this patient group. A study combining data from 11 trials of different psychosocial interventions for BED found that African American individuals were twice as likely to drop from treatment as their white counterparts. However, among remaining patients, African American patients' treatment was associated with a greater reduction in eating disorder symptoms.

Extant randomized controlled studies and treatment studies have included only a small number of Asian Americans. Thus, no definitive conclusions can be drawn. In terms of cultural considerations in tailoring CBT or any other eating disorder treatment when working with Asian American patients, Smart (2010), in a case study, recommended that treatment be time limited and solution focused. The clinician needs to keep in mind that cultural beliefs, such as equating disclosure of negative information with losing face, may affect what and how information is shared by the patient during treatment. Case formulations and treatment plans should be made by including cultural influences on body image ideals and beliefs around success and achievement in different domains. In some cases, patients benefit from including a family member in treatment to provide support, reduce stigma, and address family dynamics that affect patients' engagement in treatment.

Overall, the research on evidence-based treatments with members of ethnic minority groups is scarce. To achieve multicultural competence, clinicians should a) familiarize themselves with important characteristics of their patient's culture while considering how these may apply to the family/individual they are interacting with; b) identify personal biases and assumptions that may impact clinician's delivery of treatment; c) take into consideration patients' self-conceptualization and acculturation; and d) practice flexibly while adhering to key principles of the intervention, consulting as needed when adaptions to extant protocols are made.

Males

Despite some advancements in addressing sex biases in diagnostic criteria for eating disorders—for example, removing the amenorrhea criterion for AN in DSM-5—current criteria still do not fully capture clinical features that may be unique to males presenting with eating difficulties and related concerns. Combined with extant stereotypes regarding eating disorders affecting primarily women, this likely leads to underdetection of eating difficulties in male patients (Murray et al. 2016). Moreover, males themselves are less likely to seek treatment for eating disorders, because of the impact of these stereotypes on them as well as the paucity of information/ materials geared specifically toward males (Darcy 2011; Griffiths et al. 2015).

Lifetime prevalence rates for any eating disorder in males in community samples are estimated to be between 1.2% and 6.5% (Hudson et al. 2007; Smink et al. 2014). In contrast, prevalence rates among treatment-seeking adult samples are estimated to be between 5% and 11% (Sweeting et al. 2015), with males representing as much as one-third of adolescents seeking treatment for ARFID. Indeed, research suggests that prevalence rates for both BED and ARFID are more equivalent in males and females in adult community samples. In community samples, rates of objective binge eating, excessive exercise, and dietary restraint were also fairly equivalent in men and women (Lavender et al. 2010). In inpatient treatment settings, men were most likely to carry the diagnosis of anorexia nervosa–restricting type (AN-R) and present with overexercise (up to 81%), binge eating (42.1%), and self-induced vomiting (35%; Coelho et al. 2015; Weltzin et al. 2012).

Although there are many similarities among male and female patients presenting with eating concerns, some important differences and considerations in the diagnosis and management of eating disorders should be noted. With respect to detection and diagnosis, although prevalence of eating disorders in male athletes is lower relative to prevalence in female athletes, it is higher than among males who are not athletes, particularly among males participating in weight class sports such as wrestling and sports emphasizing leanness (Joy et al. 2016). Males also frequently have a later age at onset and a greater gap between age at onset and age at first treatment episode (Carlat et al. 1997). Relative to females, males are also more likely to present with co-occurring substance use and psychotic symptoms. In males, medical management of the eating disorder should include assessment of testosterone levels, because this is an indicator of severity of malnutrition and a risk factor for bone density loss (Mehler et al. 2008).

Although it is thought that eating disorder symptoms are not substantially different in males, there are some differences in symptoms and presentations. Because of different social cultural pressures, body image concerns in males tend to focus on leanness and muscularity rather than thinness per se or the number on the scale (Murray et al. 2013). As a result, males may be more focused than females on achieving on decreasing their percentage of body fat and "building muscle" through consuming large amounts of protein, eating frequently, excessive/compulsive exercise that focuses on strength training, monitoring their macronutrient intake, and at times even eating beyond the point of fullness to facilitate increase in muscle mass (Griffiths et al. 2013; Middleman et al. 1998). Males also score lower on measures developed to capture eating and body image concerns in female patients (i.e., drive for thinness, body dissatisfaction) (Darcy and Lin 2012). Males are as likely as females to describe objective binge-eating episodes in terms of the amount of food and show a similar degree of clinical impairment, but they are less likely to endorse experiencing loss of control during these episodes or distress after (Striegel et al. 2012).

With respect to treatment, males appear to benefit from evidence-supported interventions as much as females, with similar recovery rates for males and females receiving CBT for AN and BN (Weltzin et al. 2012) and FBT for AN (Lock et al. 2010). In fact, Stoeber and Otto (2006) reported better long-term treatment outcomes in males compared with females. Poor outcome in males was related to illness duration, quality of relationship with family, number of previous treatment episodes, and sexual activity (Burns and Crisp 1984). However, it is important to note that males have traditionally been underrepresented in studies evaluating efficacy of interventions for eating disorders. As is the case when working with females, individual case formulation should drive intervention and identify and target mechanisms unique to males presenting with eating disorder. The clinician should also keep in mind aforementioned differences in presentation as well as real and perceived barriers to seeking treatment among male patients.

Sexual and Gender Minorities

Sexual minorities, including gay and bisexual men, are at increased risk for eating disorders, with research findings suggesting that single gay men are at a particularly high risk (Brown and Keel 2012; Carlat et al. 1997). Findings suggest that being bisexual or gay is a likely risk factor for disordered eating behaviors for men (Brown and Keel 2012; Morrison et al. 2004). In both community and clinical samples, men who self-identified as bisexual or gay were more likely to endorse higher levels of disordered eating (Austin et al. 2009; Feldman and Meyer 2007; Matthews-Ewald et al. 2014; Wichstrøm 2006), body dissatisfaction (Morrison et al. 2004), and drive for thinness. Single gay men may be particularly vulnerable to internalize pressure to conform to a lean muscular body ideal, because many believe that this body type is necessary to attract potential partners and to be accepted in the gay community.

Findings regarding differences in prevalence rates between heterosexual and gay/bisexual women are mixed. Whereas Morrison et al. (2004) found that being gay or bisexual did not increase or decrease risk for eating disorders, Wichstrøm (2006) reported higher levels of disordered eating in gay and bisexual women relative to their heterosexual counterparts. Moreover, using DSM-IV diagnostic criteria for eating disorders and other mental conditions, Feldman and Meyer (2010) found that gay and bisexual men with eating disorders were more likely to have an anxiety or substance abuse disorder than gay and bisexual men without eating disorders. The authors reported that gay and bisexual women with eating disorders were more likely to have symptoms that met criteria for a mood disorder relative to their counterparts without a diagnosis of an eating disorder. In their sample, the onset of the psychiatric disorder appeared to precede the onset of the eating disorder, providing support for the theory that stress associated with adversity and stigma may increase risk for a variety of psychiatric conditions and precede eating disorder onset (Meyer 2003; Ricciardelli and McCabe 2004). Despite increased risk for disordered eating behaviors in the population, there is a paucity of research looking at detection and treatment of disordered eating behaviors and eating behaviors among sexual and gender minorities.

Common Outcomes and Complications

- The length and course of illness are variable and are dependent on factors such as age at onset, length of illness prior to treatment, access to appropriate treatment, and severity of illness.

  - Some recover quickly with rapid renourishment and aggressive, subspecialty treatment provided by experts in evidence-based treatments. Young patients whose illness is identified and treated quickly have the best prognosis.

- Others may experience a waxing and waning course of symptoms and may have periods of time when they are doing well, alternating with episodes of acute deterioration.

- Still others experience a chronic course, and about 5% may die from complications of the illness. Death is often related to the medical complications of malnutrition, including cardiac dysrhythmia. However, a substantial number of deaths in patients with anorexia nervosa are due to suicide.

- Individuals with anorexia are typically ambitious and hardworking, thus many remain enrolled in school or work.

- Individuals with bulimia nervosa may experience long periods of remission but relapse under periods of stress.

- Individuals with binge-eating disorder often struggle with overweight even after recovery.

- Outcomes of avoidant restrictive food intake disorder are not yet known, though many have lifelong disorders.

Resources and Further Reading

Online Resources

Academy for Eating Disorders: www.aedweb.org
American Academy of Child and Adolescent Psychiatry:
    www.aacap.org
American Academy of Pediatrics: www.aap.org
American Psychiatric Association: www.psychiatry.org
American Psychological Association: www.apa.org
National Eating Disorders Association:
    www.nationaleatingdisorders.org
Society for Adolescent Health and Medicine: www.adolescent-health.org

Treatment

Agras WS, Robinson A: The Oxford Handbook of Eating Disorders (Oxford Library of Psychology). New York, Oxford University Press, 2018

Fairburn CG: Overcoming Binge Eating. New York, Guilford, 1995

Grilo CM, Mitchell JE: The Treatment of Eating Disorders: A Clinical Handbook. New York, Guilford, 2011

Le Grange D, Lock J: Treating Bulimia in Adolescents: A Family Based Approach. New York, Guilford, 2007

Lock J, LeGrange D: Help Your Teenager Beat an Eating Disorder, 2nd Edition. New York, Guilford, 2005

Mehler P, Andersen A: Eating Disorders: A Guide to Medical Care and Complications, 2nd Edition. Baltimore, MD, The Johns Hopkins University Press, 2010

Mitchell JE, Devlin MJ, de Zwaan M, et al: Binge-Eating Disorder: Clinical Foundations and Treatment. New York, Guilford, 2007

Safer DL, Adler S, Masson PC: The DBT Solution for Emotional Eating: A Proven Program to Break the Cycle of Bingeing and Out-of-Control Eating. New York, Guilford, 2017

Training Resources

CBT: Oxford Cognitive Therapy Centre: https://www.octc.co.uk/training

FBT: Training Institute for Child and Adolescent Eating Disorders: train2treat4ed.com

Fairburn CG: Cognitive Behavioral Therapy and Eating Disorders. New York, Guilford, 2008

Lock J, Le Grange D: Treatment Manual for Anorexia Nervosa: A Family Based Approach, 2nd Edition. New York, Guilford, 2013

Murphy R, Straebler S, Cooper Z, et al: Interpersonal psychotherapy (IPT) for the treatment of eating disorders, in Evidence Based Treatments for Eating Disorders. Edited by Dancyger IF, Fornari V. New York, Nova, 2009, pp 257–275

Safer DL, Telch CF, Chen EY: Dialectical Behavior Therapy for Binge Eating and Bulimia. New York, Guilford, 2009

References

Ágh T, Kovács G, Supina D, et al: A systematic review of the health-related quality of life and economic burdens of anorexia nervosa, bulimia nervosa, and binge eating disorder. Eat Weight Disord 21(3):353–364, 2016 26942768

Agras WS, Apple RF: Overcoming Eating Disorders: A Cognitive-Behavioral Treatment for Bulimia Nervosa and Binge Eating Disorder. Therapist Guide. San Antonio, TX, The Psychological Corporation, 1997

Agras WS, Walsh T, Fairburn CG, et al: A multicenter comparison of cognitive-behavioral therapy and interpersonal psychotherapy for bulimia nervosa. Arch Gen Psychiatry 57(5):459–466, 2000 10807486

Agras WS, Lock J, Brandt H, et al: Comparison of 2 family therapies for adolescent anorexia nervosa: a randomized parallel trial. JAMA Psychiatry 71(11):1279–1286, 2014 25250660

Akan GE, Grilo CM: Sociocultural influences on eating attitudes and behaviors, body image, and psychological functioning: a comparison of African-American, Asian-American, and Caucasian college women. Int J Eat Disord 18(2):181–187, 1995 7581421

Alegria M, Woo M, Cao Z, et al: Prevalence and correlates of eating disorders in Latinos in the United States. Int J Eat Disord 40(suppl):S15–S21, 2007 17584870

Anderluh MB, Tchanturia K, Rabe-Hesketh S, et al: Childhood obsessive-compulsive personality traits in adult women with eating disorders: defining a broader eating disorder phenotype. Am J Psychiatry 160(2):242–247, 2003 12562569

American Psychiatric Association: Diagnostic and Statistical Manual of Mental Disorders, 3rd Edition. Washington, DC, American Psychiatric Association, 1980

American Psychiatric Association: Diagnostic and Statistical Manual of Mental Disorders, 4th Edition. Washington, DC, American Psychiatric Association, 1994

American Psychiatric Association: Diagnostic and Statistical Manual of Mental Disorders, 5th Edition. Arlington, VA, American Psychiatric Association, 2013

American Psychiatric Association: Feeding and Eating Disorders: DSM-5 Selections. Arlington, VA, American Psychiatric Association, 2015

American Psychological Association: Multicultural Guidelines: An Ecological Approach to Context, Identity, and Intersectionality. Washington, DC, American Psychological Association, 2017. Available at: http://www.apa.org/about/policy/multicultural-guidelines.PDF. Accessed July 17, 2018.

Arcelus J, Mitchell AJ, Wales J, et al: Mortality rates in patients with anorexia nervosa and other eating disorders. A meta-analysis of 36 studies. Arch Gen Psychiatry 68(7):724–731, 2011 21727255

Austin SB, Ziyadeh NJ, Corliss HL, et al: Sexual orientation disparities in purging and binge eating from early to late adolescence. J Adolesc Health 45(3):238–245, 2009 19699419

Boskind-Lodahl M: Cinderella's stepsisters: a feminist perspective on anorexia nervosa. Signs (Chic Ill) 2(2):342–356, 1976

Boskind-Lodahl M, White WC Jr: The definition and treatment of bulimarexia in college women—a pilot study. J Am Coll Health Assoc 27(2):84–86, 1978 281395

Brown TA, Keel PK: Current and emerging directions in the treatment of eating disorders. Subst Abuse 6:33–61, 2012 22879753

Bruch H: Eating Disorders: Obesity, Anorexia Nervosa, and the Person Within. New York, Basic Books, 1973

Bryant-Waugh R, Kreipe RE: Avoidant/restrictive food intake disorder in DSM-5. Psychiatr Ann 42(11):402–405, 2012

Bryant-Waugh R, Markham L, Kreipe RE, et al: Feeding and eating disorders in childhood. Int J Eat Disord 43(2):98–111, 2010 20063374

Bryant-Waugh R, Nicholls D (eds): Diagnosis and Classification of Disordered Eating in Childhood. New York, Guilford, 2011

Burns T, Crisp AH: Outcome of anorexia nervosa in males. Br J Psychiatry 145:319–325, 1984 6478127

Cachelin FM, Veisel C, Barzegarnazari E, et al: Disordered eating, acculturation, and treatment-seeking in a community sample of Hispanic, Asian, black, and white women. Psychol Women Q 24(3):244–253, 2000

Carlat DJ, Camargo CA Jr, Herzog DB: Eating disorders in males: a report on 135 patients. Am J Psychiatry 154(8):1127–1132, 1997 9247400

Childress AC, Brewerton TD, Hodges EL, et al: The Kids' Eating Disorders Survey (KEDS): a study of middle school students. J Am Acad Child Adolesc Psychiatry 32(4):843–850, 1993 8340308

Chui W, Safer DL, Bryson SW, et al: A comparison of ethnic groups in the treatment of bulimia nervosa. Eat Behav 8(4):485–491, 2007 17950937

Coelho JS, Kumar A, Kilvert M, et al: Male youth with eating disorders: clinical and medical characteristics of a sample of inpatients. Eat Disord 23(5):455–461, 2015 25826290

Cotton MA, Ball C, Robinson P: Four simple questions can help screen for eating disorders. J Gen Intern Med 18(1):53–56, 2003 12534764

Darcy A: Eating disorders in adolescent males: an critical examination of five common assumptions. Adolesc Psychiatry 1(4):307–312, 2011

Darcy AM, Lin IH: Are we asking the right questions? A review of assessment of males with eating disorders. Eat Disord 20(5):416–426, 2012 22985238

Dohm FA, Striegel-Moore RH, Wilfley DE, et al: Self-harm and substance use in a community sample of black and white women with binge eating disorder or bulimia nervosa. Int J Eat Disord 32(4):389–400, 2002 12386904

Doyle AC, McLean C, Washington BN, et al: Are single-parent families different from two-parent families in the treatment of adolescent bulimia nervosa using family based treatment? Int J Eat Disord 42(2):153–157, 2009 18720474

Fairburn CG, Cooper Z, Shafran R: Cognitive behaviour therapy for eating disorders: a "transdiagnostic" theory and treatment. Behav Res Ther 41(5):509–528, 2002 12711261

Fairburn CG, Cooper Z, Shafran R: Enhanced cognitive behavioral therapy for eating disorders ("CBT-E"): an overview, in Cognitive Behavioral Therapy and Eating Disorders. Edited by Fairburn CG. New York, Guilford, 2008, pp 23–34

Faith MS: Development of child taste and food preferences: the role of exposure, in The Oxford Handbook of Eating Disorders. Edited by Agras WS. New York, Oxford University Press, 2010, pp 137–147

Feldman MB, Meyer IH: Eating disorders in diverse lesbian, gay, and bisexual populations. Int J Eat Disord 40(3):218–226, 2007 17262818

Feldman MB, Meyer IH: Comorbidity and age of onset of eating disorders in gay men, lesbians, and bisexuals. Psychiatry Res 180(2–3):126–131, 2010 20483473

Fitzpatrick KK, Moye A, Rienecke R, et al: Adolescent focused therapy for adolescents with anorexia nervosa. J Contemp Psychother 40(1):31–39, 2009

Fitzpatrick KK, Forsberg SE, Colborn D: Family-based therapy for avoidant restrictive food intake disorder: families facing food neophobias, in Family Therapy for Adolescent Eating and Weight Disorders: New Applications. Edited by Loeb K, Le Grange D, Lock J. New York, Routledge, 2015, pp 256–276

Franko DL, Becker AE, Thomas JJ, et al: Cross-ethnic differences in eating disorder symptoms and related distress. Int J Eat Disord 40(2):156–164, 2007 17080449

Franko DL, Thompson-Brenner H, Thompson DR, et al: Racial/ethnic differences in adults in randomized clinical trials of binge eating disorder. J Consult Clin Psychol 80(2):186–195, 2012 22201327

Garner DM, Olmsted MP, Bohr Y, et al: The eating attitudes test: psychometric features and clinical correlates. Psychol Med 12(4):871–878, 1982 6961471

Garner DM, Olmstead MP, Polivy J: Development and validation of a multidimensional eating disorder inventory for anorexia nervosa and bulimia. Int J Eat Disord 2(2):15–34, 1983

George JBE, Franko DL: Cultural issues in eating pathology and body image among children and adolescents. J Pediatr Psychol 35(3):231–242, 2010 19703916

Gordon KH, Castro Y, Sitnikov L, et al: Cultural body shape ideals and eating disorder symptoms among White, Latina, and Black college women. Cultur Divers Ethnic Minor Psychol 16(2):135–143, 2010 20438151

Gowers SG, Clark A, Roberts C, et al: Clinical effectiveness of treatments for anorexia nervosa in adolescents: randomised controlled trial. Br J Psychiatry 191(5):427–435, 2007 17978323

Grabe S, Hyde JS: Ethnicity and body dissatisfaction among women in the United States: a meta-analysis. Psychol Bull 132(4):622–640, 2006 16822170

Griffiths S, Murray SB, Touyz S: Disordered eating and the muscular ideal. J Eat Disord 1(1):15, 2013 24999396

Griffiths S, Mond JM, Li Z, et al: Self-stigma of seeking treatment and being male predict an increased likelihood of having an undiagnosed eating disorder. Int J Eat Disord 48(6):775–778, 2015 26052695

Grilo CM: Psychological and behavioral treatments for binge-eating disorder. J Clin Psychiatry 78 (suppl 1):20–24, 2017 28125175

Gull W: Anorexia nervosa (apepsia hysterica, anorexia hysterica). Transactions of the Clinical Society of London 7:222–228, 1874

Halmi KA, Agras WS, Mitchell J, et al: Relapse predictors of patients with bulimia nervosa who achieved abstinence through cognitive behavioral therapy. Arch Gen Psychiatry 59(12):1105–1109, 2002 12470126

Halmi KA, Bellace D, Berthod S, et al: An examination of early childhood perfectionism across anorexia nervosa subtypes. Int J Eat Disord 45(6):800–807, 2012 22488115

Hatmaker G: Boys with eating disorders. J Sch Nurs 21(6):329–332, 2005 16419341

Hay P: A systematic review of evidence for psychological treatments in eating disorders: 2005–2012. Int J Eat Disord 46(5):462–469, 2013 23658093

Hay PJ, Claudino AM: Clinical psychopharmacology of eating disorders: a research update. Int J Neuropsychopharmacol 15(2):209–222, 2012 21439105

Hay PP, Bacaltchuk J, Stefano S, et al: Psychological treatments for bulimia nervosa and binging. Cochrane Database Syst Rev (4):CD000562, 2009 19821271

Hay PJ, Touyz S, Sud R: Treatment for severe and enduring anorexia nervosa: a review. Aust N Z J Psychiatry 46(12):1136–1144, 2012 22696548

Hoek HW, van Hoeken D: Review of the prevalence and incidence of eating disorders. Int J Eat Disord 34(4):383–396, 2003 14566926

Hoek HW, van Harten PN, Hermans KM, et al: The incidence of anorexia nervosa on Curaçao. Am J Psychiatry 162(4):748–752, 2005 15800148

Hudson JI, Hiripi E, Pope HG Jr, et al: The prevalence and correlates of eating disorders in the National Comorbidity Survey Replication. Biol Psychiatry 61(3):348–358, 2007 16815322

Jones DC, Vigfusdottir TH, Lee Y: Body image and the appearance culture among adolescent girls and boys: an examination of friend conversations, peer criticism, appearance magazines, and the internalization of appearance ideals. J Adolesc Res 19(3):323–339, 2004

Joy E, Kussman A, Nattiv A: 2016 update on eating disorders in athletes: A comprehensive narrative review with a focus on clinical assessment and management. Br J Sports Med 50(3):154–162, 2016 26782763

Keys A, Brozek J, Henschel A: The Biology of Human Starvation. Minneapolis, University of Minnesota Press, 1950

Kreipe RE, Palomaki A: Beyond picky eating: avoidant/restrictive food intake disorder. Curr Psychiatry Rep 14(4):421–431, 2012 22665043

Lavender JM, De Young KP, Anderson DA: Eating Disorder Examination Questionnaire (EDE-Q): norms for undergraduate men. Eat Behav 11(2):119–121, 2010 20188296

Le Grange D, Lock J: Bulimia nervosa in adolescents: treatment, eating pathology, and comorbidity. S Afr Psychiatry Rev 5:19–22, 2002

Le Grange D, Lock J: Treating Bulimia in Adolescence. New York, Guilford, 2007

Le Grange D, Lock J, Agras WS, et al: Randomized clinical trial of family-based treatment and cognitive-behavioral therapy for adolescent bulimia nervosa. J Am Acad Child Adolesc Psychiatry 54(11):886–894, 2015 26506579

Lee S: Self-starvation in context: towards a culturally sensitive understanding of anorexia nervosa. Soc Sci Med 41(1):25–36, 1995 7667670

Ling YL, Rascati KL, Pawaskar M: Direct and indirect costs among patients with binge-eating disorder in the United States. Int J Eat Disord 50(5):523–532, 2017 27862132

Lock J: Trying to fit square pegs in round holes: eating disorders in males. J Adolesc Health 44(2):99–100, 2008 19167655

Lock J: Treatment of adolescent eating disorders: progress and challenges. Minerva Psichiatr 51(3):207–216, 2010 21532979

Lock J: Update on evidence-based psychosocial treatments for eating disorders in children and adolescents. J Clin Child Adolesc Psychol 44(5):707–721, 2015 25580937

Lock J, Le Grange D: Family based treatment of eating disorders. Int J Eat Disord 37(suppl):S64–S67, discussion S87–S89, 2005 15852323

Lock J, Le Grange D: Treatment Manual for Anorexia Nervosa: A Family Based Approach. New York, Guilford, 2013

Lock J, Le Grange D, Agras WS, et al: Randomized clinical trial comparing family based treatment with adolescent-focused individual therapy for adolescents with anorexia nervosa. Arch Gen Psychiatry 67(10):1025–1032, 2010 20921118

Marcus MD, Kalarchian MA: Binge eating in children and adolescents. Int J Eat Disord 34(suppl):S47–S57, 2003 12900986

Marques L, Alegria M, Becker AE, et al: Comparative prevalence, correlates of impairment, and service utilization for eating disorders across US ethnic groups: Implications for reducing ethnic disparities in health care access for eating disorders. Int J Eat Disord 44(5):412–420, 2011 20665700

Matthews-Ewald MR, Zullig KJ, Ward RM: Sexual orientation and disordered eating behaviors among self-identified male and female college students. Eat Behav 15(3):441–444, 2014 25064296

McElroy SL: Pharmacologic treatments for binge-eating disorder. J Clin Psychiatry 78(suppl 1):14–19, 2017 28125174

McKenzie JM, Joyce PR: Hospitalization for anorexia nervosa. Int J Eat Disord 11(3):235–241, 1992

Mehler PS, Sabel AL, Watson T, et al: High risk of osteoporosis in male patients with eating disorders. Int J Eat Disord 41(7):666–672, 2008 18528874

Meyer IH: Prejudice, social stress, and mental health in lesbian, gay, and bisexual populations: conceptual issues and research evidence. Psychol Bull 129(5):674–697, 2003 12956539

Middleman AB, Vazquez I, Durant RH: Eating patterns, physical activity, and attempts to change weight among adolescents. J Adolesc Health 22(1):37–42, 1998 9436065

Mintz LB, Kashubeck S: Body image and disordered eating among Asian American and Caucasian college students: an examination of race and gender differences. Psychol Women Q 23(4):781–796, 1999

Morgan JF, Reid F, Lacey JH: The SCOFF questionnaire: assessment of a new screening tool for eating disorders. BMJ 319(7223):1467–1468, 1999 10582927

Morrison MA, Morrison TG, Sager CL: Does body satisfaction differ between gay men and lesbian women and heterosexual men and women? A meta-analytic review. Body Image 1(2):127–138, 2004 18089146

Morton R: Phthisiologia: Or, a Treatise of Consumptions. London, Smith & Walford, 1694

Murray SB, Rieger E, Karlov L, et al: Masculinity and femininity in the divergence of male body image concerns. J Eat Disord 1:11, 2013 24999393

Murray SB, Griffiths S, Mond JM: Evolving eating disorder psychopathology: conceptualising muscularity-oriented disordered eating. Br J Psychiatry 208(5):414–415, 2016 27143005

Nicholls D, Chater R, Lask B: Children into DSM don't go: a comparison of classification systems for eating disorders in childhood and early adolescence. Int J Eat Disord 28(3):317–324, 2000 10942918

Nicholls D, Randall D, Randall L, et al: Selective eating: symptom disorder or normal variant? Clin Child Psychol Psychiatry 6(2):257–270, 2001

Passi VA, Bryson SW, Lock J: Assessment of eating disorders in adolescents with anorexia nervosa: self-report questionnaire versus interview. Int J Eat Disord 33(1):45–54, 2003 12474198

Peat CM, Berkman ND, Lohr KN, et al: Comparative effectiveness of treatments for binge-eating disorder: Systematic review and network meta-analysis. Eur Eat Disord Rev 25(5):317–328, 2017 28467032

Perez M, Plasencia M: Psychological perspectives on ethnic minority eating behavior and obesity, in Social Issues in Living Color: Challenges and Solutions From the Perspective of Ethnic Minority Psychology, Vol 3. Edited by Blume AW. Santa Barbara, CA, Praeger, 2016, pp 103–128

Perez M, Ohrt TK, Hoek HW: Prevalence and treatment of eating disorders among Hispanics/Latino Americans in the United States. Curr Opin Psychiatry 29(6):378–382, 2016 27648780

Pike KM, Wilfley D, Hilbert A, et al: Antecedent life events of binge-eating disorder. Psychiatry Res 142(1):19–29, 2006 16713629

Pote H, Stratton P, Cottrell D, et al: Systemic Family Therapy Manual. Leeds, UK, Leeds Family Therapy and Research Centre, University of Leeds, 2001. Available at: https://medhealth.leeds.ac.uk/download/665/leeds_systemic_family_therapy_manual. Accessed August 1, 2001.

Reyes-Rodríguez ML, Bulik C: Toward a cultural adaptation of eating disorders treatment for Latinos in United States. Mexican Journal of Eating Disorders 1:27–35, 2010

Reyes-Rodríguez ML, Franko DL, Matos-Lamourt A, et al: Eating disorder symptomatology: prevalence among Latino college freshmen students. J Clin Psychol 66(6):666–679, 2010 20455253

Reyes-Rodríguez ML, Bulik CM, Hamer RM, et al: Promoviendo una alimentación saludable (PAS) design and methods: engaging Latino families in eating disorder treatment. Contemp Clin Trials 35(1):52–61, 2013 23376815

Reyes-Rodríguez ML, Gulisano M, Silva Y, et al: "Las penas con pan duelen menos": the role of food and culture in Latinas with disordered eating behaviors. Appetite 100:102–109, 2016 26911262

Ricciardelli LA, McCabe MP: A biopsychosocial model of disordered eating and the pursuit of muscularity in adolescent boys. Psychol Bull 130(2):179–205, 2004 14979769

Rieger E, Van Buren DJ, Bishop M, et al: An eating disorder-specific model of interpersonal psychotherapy (IPT-ED): causal pathways and treatment implications. Clin Psychol Rev 30(4):400–410, 2010 20227151

Russell G: Bulimia nervosa: an ominous variant of anorexia nervosa. Psychol Med 9(3):429–448, 1979 482466

Russell G: The history of bulimia nervosa, in Handbook of Treatment for Eating Disorders. Edited by Garner DM, Garfinkel P. New York, Guilford, 1997, pp 11–24

Safer DL, Telch CF, Agras WS: Dialectical behavior therapy for bulimia nervosa. Am J Psychiatry 158(4):632–634, 2001 11282700

Safer DL, Couturier J, Lock J, et al: Dialectical behavior therapy modified for adolescent binge eating disorders: a case report. Cognitive Behavioral Practice 14(2):157–167, 2007

Safer DC, Telch F, Chen EY: Dialectical Behavior Therapy for Binge Eating and Bulimia. New York, Guilford, 2009

Safer DL, Robinson AH, Jo B: Outcome from a randomized controlled trial of group therapy for binge eating disorder: comparing dialectical behavior therapy adapted for binge eating to an active comparison group therapy. Behav Ther 41(1):106–120, 2010 20171332

Saraf M: Holy anorexia and anorexia nervosa: society and concept of disease. Pharos Alpha Omega Alpha Honor Med Soc 61(4):2–4, 1998 9884606

Shea M, Cachelin F, Uribe L, et al: Cultural adaptation of a cognitive behavior therapy guided self-help program for Mexican American women with binge eating disorders. J Couns Dev 90(3):308–318, 2012 23645969

Sinha S, Warfa N: Treatment of eating disorders among ethnic minorities in Western settings: a systematic review. Psychiatr Danub 25(suppl 2):S295–S299, 2013 23995197

Smart R: Treating Asian American women with eating disorders: multicultural competency and empirically supported treatment. Eat Disord 18(1):58–73, 2010 20390608

Smink FR, van Hoeken D, Hoek HW: Epidemiology of eating disorders: incidence, prevalence and mortality rates. Curr Psychiatry Rep 14(4):406–414, 2012 22644309

Smink FRE, van Hoeken D, Oldehinkel AJ, et al: Prevalence and severity of DSM-5 eating disorders in a community cohort of adolescents. Int J Eat Disord 47(6):610–619, 2014 24903034

Soh NL, Touyz SW, Surgenor LJ: Eating and body image disturbances across cultures: a review. Eur Eat Disord Rev 14(1):54–65, 2006

Sonneville KR, Calzo JP, Horton NJ, et al: Body satisfaction, weight gain and binge eating among overweight adolescent girls. Int J Obes 36(7):944–949, 2012 22565419

Stice E, Agras WS: Predicting onset and cessation of bulimic behaviors during adolescence. Behav Ther 29(2):257–276, 1998

Stoeber J, Otto K: Positive conceptions of perfectionism: approaches, evidence, challenges. Pers Soc Psychol Rev 10(4):295–319, 2006 17201590

Striegel RH, Bedrosian R, Wang C, Schwartz S: Why men should be included in research on binge eating: results from a comparison of psychosocial impairment in men and women. Int J Eat Disord 45(2):233–240, 2012 22031213

Striegel-Moore RH, Dohm FA, Kraemer HC, et al: Eating disorders in white and black women. Am J Psychiatry 160(7):1326–1331, 2003 12832249

Stunkard AJ: Eating patterns and obesity. Psychiatr Q 33:284–295, 1959 13835451

Swanson SA, Crow SJ, Le Grange D, et al: Prevalence and correlates of eating disorders in adolescents. Results from the national comorbidity survey replication adolescent supplement. Arch Gen Psychiatry 68(7):714–723, 2011 21383252

Sweeting H, Walker L, MacLean A, et al: Prevalence of eating disorders in males: a review of rates reported in academic research and UK mass media. Int J Mens Health 14(2): 2015 26290657

Taylor JY, Caldwell CH, Baser RE, et al: Prevalence of eating disorders among Blacks in the National Survey of American Life. Int J Eat Disord 40(suppl):S10–S14, 2007 17879287

Telch CF, Stice E: Psychiatric comorbidity in women with binge eating disorder: prevalence rates from a non-treatment-seeking sample. J Consult Clin Psychol 66(5):768–776, 1998 9803695

Telch CF, Agras WS, Linehan MM: Group dialectical behavior therapy for binge-eating disorder: a preliminary, uncontrolled trial. Behav Ther 31(3):569–582, 2000

Telch CF, Agras WS, Linehan MM: Dialectical behavior therapy for binge eating disorder. J Consult Clin Psychol 69(6):1061–1065, 2001 11777110

Thoma H: Anorexia Nervosa. New York, International Universities Press, 1967

Thomas JJ, Lawson EA, Micali N, et al: Avoidant/restrictive food intake disorder: a three-dimensional model of neurobiology with implications for etiology and treatment. Curr Psychiatry Rep 19(8):54, 2017

Trace SE, Baker JH, Peñas-Lledó E, et al: The genetics of eating disorders. Annu Rev Clin Psychol 9:589–620, 2013 23537489

Treasure J, Russell G: The case for early intervention in anorexia nervosa: theoretical exploration of maintaining factors. Br J Psychiatry 199(1):5–7, 2011 21719874

van Son GE, van Hoeken D, Bartelds AI, et al: Time trends in the incidence of eating disorders: a primary care study in the Netherlands. Int J Eat Disord 39(7):565–569, 2006 16791852

Vocks S, Tuschen-Caffier B, Pietrowsky R, et al: Meta-analysis of the effectiveness of psychological and pharmacological treatments for binge eating disorder. Int J Eat Disord 43(3):205–217, 2010 19402028

Watson HJ, Bulik CM: Update on the treatment of anorexia nervosa: review of clinical trials, practice guidelines and emerging interventions. Psychol Med 43(12):2477–2500, 2013 23217606

Weltzin TE, Cornella-Carlson T, Fitzpatrick ME, et al: Treatment issues and outcomes for males with eating disorders. Eat Disord 20(5):444–459, 2012 22985241

Wichstrøm L: Sexual orientation as a risk factor for bulimic symptoms. Int J Eat Disord 39(6):448–453, 2006 16634052

Wilfley DE, Welch RR, Stein RI, et al: A randomized comparison of group cognitive-behavioral therapy and group interpersonal psychotherapy for the treatment of overweight individuals with binge-eating disorder. Arch Gen Psychiatry 59(8):713–721, 2002 12150647

Yokoyama K: The double binds of our bodies: multiculturally-informed feminist therapy considerations for body image and eating disorders among Asian American women. Women Ther 30(3–4):177–192, 2007

Zipfel S, Wild B, Gross G, et al: Focal psychodynamic therapy, cognitive behaviour therapy, and optimised treatment as usual in outpatients with anorexia nervosa (ANTOP study): randomised controlled trial. Lancet 383(9912):127–137, 2014 24131861

Chapter 2

Anorexia Nervosa

Jennifer Derenne, M.D.
James Lock, M.D., Ph.D.

Introduction

Anorexia nervosa (AN) is a severe, biologically based illness that sometimes has a chronic relapsing and remitting course. It is the mental health disorder with the highest mortality rate of all psychiatric illnesses aside from the substance use disorders (Birmingham et al. 2005; Crow et al. 2009). Death is generally secondary to the consequences of malnutrition, particularly cardiovascular dysrhythmia (Jáuregui-Garrido and Jáuregui-Lobera 2012). However, a significant proportion of patients die by suicide (Lock 2015). Although once thought to be primarily a disorder of affluent white teenage girls, we now know that AN affects individuals across the lifespan and gender spectrum, as well as all ethnic and socioeconomic backgrounds.

The pathognomonic feature of AN is significant concern about body weight and shape, which drives behaviors that lead to weight loss or failure to meet expected growth requirements in children and adolescents. Typically, individuals with AN experience a disturbance in how they perceive their bodies and may believe that they are overweight or need to lose weight even when presented with evidence that they are underweight or medically compromised because of malnutrition. Others may deny body image concerns but continue to have difficulty modifying their behaviors to minimize exercise and increase nutritional intake. DSM-5 (American Psychiatric Association 2013) employs modified language that removes potentially stigmatizing language, eliminates a specific weight cutpoint for adolescent AN, and removes the diagnostic requirement for amenorrhea. This is important because males do not menstruate and the use of contraception may cause withdrawal bleeding.

The medical complications of eating disorders are widespread and affect every organ system in the body (Golden et al. 2015). For this reason, the treatment of AN requires regular follow-up with clinicians who are familiar and experienced with the medical monitoring of eating disorders. Mental health treatment should generally be delivered by a provider with expertise in the evidence-based treatments for AN. With rare exceptions, psychotropic medications are not indicated in the treatment of AN itself, because no psychiatric medicines have been shown to be effective for the disorder (Golden and Attia 2011). However, psychotropics are commonly used to treat premorbid and comorbid psychiatric conditions, such as mood or anxiety disorders. At the same time, it is important to remember that the consequences of malnutrition can mimic the neurovegetative symptoms of depression, and the act of eating and fear of weight gain can trigger anxiety in patients with AN; these symptoms are generally part of AN and best treated with safe renourishment and behavioral strategies for managing distress and normalizing and regulating eating patterns. Registered dietitians sometimes provide education to patients and parents requesting consultation about nutrition needs. If several clinicians are involved in the care of the patient, as is usually necessary with AN, all team members must work together collaboratively and communicate closely in order to present a unified set of recommendations to the patient and family.

Key Diagnostic Checklist

❏ Inadequate nutrition intake relative to energy needs

❏ Significantly low weight or failure to attain expected growth

❏ Intense fear of weight gain or becoming overweight, or behavior that interferes with weight gain

❏ Disturbance in perception of weight or shape, undue influence of weight and shape on self-evaluation, or inability to recognize the severity of low weight

❏ *Restricting subtype:* achieving weight loss through restriction and/or excessive exercise

❏ *Binge-eating/purging subtype:* engaging in recurrent binge eating or purging (inducing vomiting or use of laxatives, diuretics, emetics) over the preceding 3 months

Diagnostic Rule Outs

Medical

Typically, patients are aware and concerned about weight loss, are trying to increase intake and do not experience negative body image.

- Malignancy
- HIV/AIDS
- Hyperthyroidism
- Gastrointestinal disorders: inflammatory bowel disease, celiac sprue
- Rheumatological illness: systemic lupus erythematosus

Psychiatric

- *Avoidant/restrictive food intake disorder.* Patients with avoidant restrictive food intake disorders do not express body image concerns or desire to lose weight. Difficulty eating is generally related to physical discomfort, anxiety, or longstanding food preferences.
- *Bulimia nervosa.* Patients with bulimia nervosa engage in recurrent binge eating and compensatory purging behaviors. They are often concerned about weight and shape, but weight is generally normal or above normal.
- *Major depressive disorder.* Loss of appetite is a neurovegetative symptom associated with depression and may result in weight loss. However, patients with major depressive disorder do not generally experience body image concerns and do not want to lose weight.
- *Schizophrenia.* Psychosis can result in inadequate nutrition intake due to paranoia or disorganization. However, patients do not have negative body image and do not wish to lose weight.
- *Substance use disorders.* Substance use disorders may lead to weight loss secondary to poor nutritional intake, related to either decreased appetite or chronic intoxication. There is typically no body image disturbance. Some drugs, such as stimulants and cocaine, may be abused in the setting of anorexia nervosa with the intent to decrease appetite and encourage weight loss.
- *Anxiety disorders (generalized anxiety, social anxiety disorder) and obsessive-compulsive and related disorders*

(obsessive-compulsive disorder, body dysmorphic disorder). Anxiety may lead to loss of appetite and difficulty eating. Examples include worries about eating in front of other people, engaging in elaborate food rituals, or the belief that a body part is misshapen or too big.

Epidemiology and Risk Factors

- Anorexia nervosa has a prevalence of 0.5%–1.5% in young women (Smink et al. 2014). Current estimates suggest that the ratio of females to males is 10:1 (Hatmaker 2005; Lock 2008).
- Anorexia nervosa typically arises in a "perfect storm" of biopsychosocial factors that may make an individual vulnerable. There is generally not one precipitating factor.

  - *Biological factors.* There is a genetic vulnerability in first-degree relatives of individuals with eating disorders. Weight loss may precipitate disordered eating; hormonal changes associated with puberty and later life may also confer some risk.
  - *Psychological factors.* Perfectionistic, harm avoidant, and self-doubting temperaments increase risk (Anderluh et al. 2003). Separations and transitions, as well as stressful life events such as moving, taking on a new job, or dealing with the loss of a loved one, may increase risk.
  - *Social and environmental factors.* Societal preoccupation with thinness; dieting (Jones 2004); or participation in activities that involve a desired body type or weight classes (such as wrestling, rowing, gymnastics, figure skating, or ballet) increases risk.

Common Comorbidities

Medical

- Gastroparesis
- Constipation
- Amenorrhea, sexual dysfunction, infertility
- Sick euthyroid

- Pancytopenia
- Bradycardia, prolonged QTc, dysrhythmia
- Osteoporosis
- Electrolyte abnormalities—potassium may be low from purging
- Refeeding syndrome—phosphate and magnesium levels may decrease because of shifts related to renourishment
- Gastroesophageal reflux disease
- Vitamin D deficiency

Psychiatric

- Mood disorders (particularly depression and bipolar disorder)—care must be taken to screen and monitor for suicidal ideation as many patients with eating disorders die by suicide.
- Anxiety disorders
- Obsessive-compulsive disorder
- Substance use disorders
- Personality disorders

Assessment

The first step in determining a treatment plan for a patient with AN is to make an appropriate diagnosis through a comprehensive medical and psychiatric assessment (Figure 2–1). The medical evaluation should be conducted by a provider familiar with assessing the medical complications of malnutrition. Vital signs should be reviewed, including orthostatic blood pressures in the lying and standing positions. Body mass index (BMI) should be calculated to determine the degree of weight loss and malnutrition (in children and adolescents, the percentage of median BMI for age, height, and gender is used to determine the degree of malnutrition). A full physical examination should be conducted, with care taken to fully evaluate the cardiovascular system. An electrocardiogram is useful to document bradycardia as well as to measure the QTc interval. Finally, laboratory studies are needed to be sure that elec-

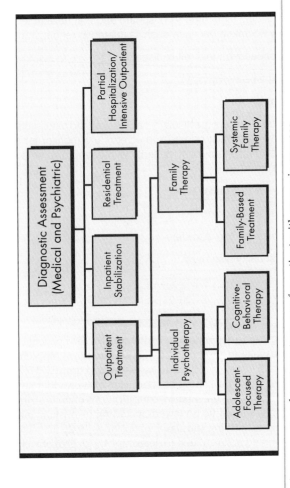

FIGURE 2–1.   Assessment and treatment process for patient with anorexia nervosa.

trolytes are within the normal range, as well as to screen for other medical conditions that may lead to unexplained weight loss (Medicine 1995).

The psychiatric evaluation includes a complete history of the patient's symptoms and behaviors. It is important to have a sense of the weight history, personal and family attitudes about weight and shape, and a full understanding of the nature and frequency of restrictive eating, binge eating, purging, and exercise patterns. Especially with children and adolescents, collateral sources should be interviewed to obtain a complete history; these may include parents, teachers, and coaches. Speaking to significant others and family members can be very useful when assessing adults as well (Lock 2015; Yager 2006). In addition, it is important to complete a full psychiatric review of symptoms to determine whether there are comorbid conditions, such as mood or anxiety disorders, that may complicate treatment. Given that malnutrition can mimic many of the neurovegetative symptoms of depression, it is necessary for the clinician to carefully establish the timeline of symptom development. Mood and anxiety related to malnutrition is likely best treated with renourishment, while premorbid mood and anxiety disorders may require psychotropic medications and/or additional psychotherapeutic interventions. Because many deaths in patients with AN are due to completed suicide, it is essential that the clinician perform a comprehensive safety assessment.

Clinical Presentation

Suzie

Suzie is a 13-year-old female whose parents bring her to the pediatrician with concerns about **weight loss** and changes in behavior. She has always tracked around the 90th percentile for weight. At her well-child visit last year, the pediatrician made a comment about the need to eat healthfully and stay active so that she did not develop the problems with high cholesterol that are common in her family. Since that time, her parents have noted that she has increased her activity while decreasing her intake. Initially they thought it was fine for her to make an effort to eat fruits and vegetables and to limit her intake of junk food. However, as she began to lose weight, her peers and teachers commented that she "looked really good," and this seemed to push her to make even more **drastic dietary restrictions**. Suzie has progressively narrowed her intake to the point that she is now only eating steamed vegetables and egg whites at each meal. She refuses to drink anything other than water, and states that she no longer "likes" sugar, dairy, meat, and foods containing gluten. She also believes that these foods make her feel sick. Parents have been trying to encourage her to eat more, but she refuses. She has taken up baking and now makes all sorts of delicious treats for the family, but she refuses to eat anything that she makes.

In addition to her **strict dieting**, Suzie now **exercises at least an hour each day**. This exercise includes running at the local high school track and doing crunches, pushups, and planks. She becomes highly irritated if she thinks that she may not be able to fit in a workout. Suzie's parents note that while she used to play with the other girls in the neighborhood, she is now isolating herself at home. She stands while doing her homework and while she eats her meals.

Suzie's parents have noticed that Suzie spends a long time in the bathroom after meals, but they have listened at the door and do not think that she is vomiting. She denies use of laxatives, emetics, diuretics, stimulants, or diet pills. Suzie says that she knows that she has lost a lot of weight (more than 20 pounds), but she feels as though she could work on being "healthier." She states that she spends a lot of time looking at herself in the mirror after meals because she is **worried that the food she ate is turning to fat**. She stopped menstruating 4 months ago. Suzie is always cold and wears a baggy sweatshirt even when it is warm outside.

Suzie and her parents acknowledge that she is more fatigued lately and needs to nap after school, even though she slept 8 hours the night before. She becomes annoyed with her parents when they encourage her to eat and has become more easily irritated in general, which is out of character for her. Her concentration and focus have been unchanged, however. Despite not feeling like herself, she earned all A's on her report card last term while also being involved in student council, violin lessons, and chess club. Her parents state, "She always gives 110%."

Evidence-Based Outpatient Treatments for Anorexia Nervosa

Adults

Cognitive-behavioral therapy (Fairburn et al. 2008)—Level 3 (possibly efficacious)

Focal psychodynamic individual therapy (Zipfel et al. 2014)—Level 3 (possibly efficacious)

Children and Adolescents

Family-based treatment (Lock and Le Grange 2013)—Level 1 (established treatment)

Adolescent-focused treatment (Fitzpatrick et al. 2009)—Level 2 (possibly efficacious)

Systemic family therapy (Agras et al. 2014)—Level 3 (probably efficacious)

Cognitive-behavioral therapy (Gowers et al. 2007)—Level 4 (experimental treatment)

Treatment Settings

After the initial assessment is complete, the evaluating providers can make a recommendation on the appropriate venue for initial treatment. Generally, the first decision point involves the choice between outpatient treatment and a higher level of care. These are described at length in the next section. If the patient is medically unstable, inpatient hospitalization is likely needed. If suicide is a concern, inpatient psychiatric hospitalization might be required (Yager 2006). Children and adolescents who are medically stable for outpatient treatment are generally best served by a family-based treatment (FBT) approach, whereas adults who do not live with parents may do better with a more individualized approach. It is important to acknowledge, however, that young adults, in particular, often benefit from parent involvement in treatment, even when they are older than 18 years of age.

For patients of any age, the most important initial interventions focus on renourishment and behavioral change. Medical stabilization of heart rates and blood pressures and weight restoration are top priority (Mehler and Brown 2015). This is typically accomplished by increasing nutrition while limiting activity; in a hospital setting, this would involve placing the patient on bed rest while increasing intake in a safe and monitored fashion. Depending on the degree of malnutrition, clinicians need to make a decision about where to start renourishment. While conventional wisdom dictates that it is important to "start low and go slow" to avoid possible refeeding syndrome, recent studies have suggested that it is safe to start at higher calorie levels and increase more quickly as long as laboratory studies are monitored closely so that electrolyte and phosphorus levels can be corrected quickly if they become abnormal (Skipper 2012). While many patients experience discomfort with the renourishment process due to increased volumes of foods that they are not used to eating, it is important to use the gastrointestinal tract for food and fluids. Nutritional supplement drinks can be used to replace calories from food that the patient is not willing or able to eat. If the patient refuses to drink the supplement orally and is medically unstable, nasogastric tubes can be used to keep the renourishment process on track.

During treatment for medical instability, it is important to begin to normalize and regulate eating patterns and to stop compulsive exercise. Individuals benefit from having three structured meals and two or three snacks per day spaced at appropriate intervals. This enables the patient to work on listening to hunger and satiety cues and avoid the urge to restrict eating. Regular meals and snacks help prevent binge-eating and purging behaviors as well, because eating at regular intervals prevents hunger from developing, which is often a trigger for binge eating. In the beginning, activity is generally restricted until weight is restored and vital signs have normalized. The monitoring physician may then allow a gradual return to balanced activity as long as the patient is able to take in enough nutrition to support the body's increased energy needs.

Levels of Care

- *Inpatient medical stabilization.* This level of care is necessary when the patient is severely medically ill and requires intensive medical monitoring for safe renourishment (Tables 2–1 and 2–2). This may include cardiac monitoring, frequent laboratory draws, and additional subspecialty consultation and testing for the treatment of medical sequelae of malnutrition.

- *Inpatient psychiatric.* This level of care is indicated when the patient is medically stable but is exhibiting concerning behaviors such as suicidal ideation, uncontrolled purging, or acute food refusal. Not all inpatient psychiatric units can successfully manage eating disorders because of the labor-intensive nature of monitoring meals and snacks, but some have special tracks for eating disorder patients.

- *Residential treatment center.* This level of care is appropriate when the individual is medically and psychiatrically stable but needs increased structure and support to abstain from disordered eating behaviors. Patients needing this level of care usually have failed outpatient treatment, or there is no outpatient treatment available to them locally. Patients live in the treatment setting, typically for extended periods of time (30, 60, or 90 days or more). Treatment generally includes meal support, individual psychotherapy, group psychotherapy, and family therapy as well as therapeutic outings and food challenges that are intended to help the patient practice the return to "normal" life. While people are often able to restore and maintain weight in a supervised setting, a downside of residential treatment is that many begin to fall back into old patterns and may even relapse when they leave the structured setting and return to the stresses of regular life (Brewerton and Costin 2011a, 2011b).

- *Partial hospital program (PHP).* Day hospital programs are similar to residential treatment, except that patients return home at the end of the day. This allows some time with family and permits the patient to sleep at home. Being home introduces typical environmental stresses and gives individuals an opportunity to practice recovery behaviors with the support of their team. Again, the structure and support allow individuals to restore and maintain weight, but without focusing on changing the home environment and coping behaviors, relapse is common after discharge home. Some programs operate 7 days per week, whereas others are open Monday through Friday (Herpertz-Dahlmann et al. 2014).

- *Intensive outpatient program (IOP).* This level of care is often a "stepdown" from partial hospitalization, and many programs offer both levels of care. IOP offers similar meal support and group therapy to that offered in PHPs. However, these programs typically last 3–4 hours per day during the work week. This reduced time in structured programming allows patients to return to school or work yet offers structure and support during vulnerable hours. As with PHP and

TABLE 2–1. Medical admission criteria for adolescents with anorexia nervosa

Bradycardia	Pulse < 50 BPM daytime, < 45 BPM night
Hypotension	BP < 90/45 mm Hg
Hypothermia	Temperature < 35.6°C/96°F
Orthostasis (from supine to standing position)	Pulse increases > 20 BPM
	Systolic BP decrease > 20 mm Hg
	Diastolic BP decrease > 10 mm Hg
Weight	< 75% median BMI for age and sex
Electrocardiographic abnormalities	Prolonged QTc > 460 msec, for example
Electrolyte abnormalities	Phosphorus < 3.0 mg/dL
	Potassium < 3.5 mEq/L
	Magnesium < 1.8 mg/dL
Other acute medical events	Syncope, gastrointestinal bleeding, severe dehydration, for example

Note. BMI=body mass index; BP=blood pressure; BPM=beats per minute.

residential programs, individuals often return to disordered eating patterns without the structure and support of a program in place.

- *Outpatient treatment.* Outpatient treatment typically involves appointments with a medical provider and one or two sessions per week with a psychotherapist who has experience treating eating disorders. Depending on the treatment modality employed, patients or parents may also consult with a dietitian for assistance with meal planning. If psychotropic medications are being used to manage comorbid psychiatric conditions, a psychiatrist will also be involved. It is important that the treatment team communicate closely to make sure that all providers are giving consistent recommendations to patients and their families.

TABLE 2–2. Medical admission criteria for adults with anorexia nervosa

Weight	< 85% of individually estimated healthy body weight
Bradycardia	Pulse < 40 BPM
Hypotension	BP < 90/60 mm Hg
Hypothermia	Temperature < 36.1°C/97°F
Electrolyte imbalance	Potassium < 3 mEq/L
Hypoglycemia	Glucose < 60 mg/dL
Other acute medical events	Dehydration; poorly controlled diabetes; hepatic, renal, cardiovascular organ compromise requiring acute treatment

Note. BP=blood pressure; BPM=beats per minute.

Treatments

Family-Based Treatment

FBT (Lock and Le Grange 2013) is a three-phase treatment that has the most data to date supporting its use in treating adolescent AN. Six randomized controlled trials have evaluated family therapy for adolescents with AN (Lock et al. 2006; Lock et al. 2010). The findings from these studies and a meta-analysis of randomized controlled trials support the view that FBT is a Level 1 empirically supported treatment for adolescents with AN (Lock et al. 2015).

The patient, parents, and siblings attend weekly family therapy sessions focused on increasing intake and minimizing activity. FBT consists of between 10 and 20 family meetings over a 6- to 12-month treatment course. FBT empowers parents to take charge of the weight restoration of their child, disrupting symptoms of self-starvation and overexercise. Once the child is able to eat independently without parental supervision and has reached a normal weight, the treatment briefly focuses on developmental issues of adolescence.

In the first phase, parents are tasked with planning, preparing, serving, and observing all meals and snacks, with the goal of helping the patient restore weight. When weight restoration has been achieved, the second phase focuses on gradually transitioning decision making about eating back to the patient in an age-appropriate manner, but the parents continue to monitor eating and step in if needed to prevent relapse. The third phase of treatment begins only after the symptoms of AN are fully abated. The treatment shifts to focus on age-appropriate independence as well as discussion of normal adolescent life issues and relapse prevention (Forsberg and Lock 2015).

Systemic Family Therapy

Systemic family therapy (SyFT) is a manualized treatment that is delivered over the course of 16 sessions and focuses on relationships and interactions between family members rather than on food and eating. Data supporting systemic family approaches to AN are more limited than for FBT, and SyFT is considered a Level 3 (i.e., possibly efficacious) treatment. One study conducted at a university-affiliated clinical program in Paris compared posthospitalization outcome for adolescents with AN who received treatment as usual or treatment as usual plus a form of SyFT (Godart et al. 2012). Family therapy sessions lasted 1.5 hours and occurred at 3- to 4-week intervals for 18 months. The 60 female participants in the study (30 per group) ranged from 13 and 19 years of age. There were significant differences between randomized groups, but among completers, participants who received treatment as usual plus family therapy had better outcomes. A more rigorous comparison test of SyFT compared it with FBT in a six-site study with 167 adolescents with AN and their families participating (Agras et al. 2014). There were no differences in clinical outcomes between the groups, but FBT restored weight significantly faster, used less hospitalization, and was much less expensive.

SyFT was developed and manualized by researchers at Leeds University as a model of treatment based on a family systems model (Pote 2003). SyFT focused on identifying, understanding, and changing patterns of behavior and beliefs. By helping the family understand these patterns, the therapist helps the family to consider new or different approaches that might be healthier for the family. SyFT approaches the family as a system, by examining the ways they organize themselves as a family in terms of their different roles and relationships. There are three stages to SyFT. In the first stage, the goals are to 1) discuss therapy boundaries therapeutic structure; 2) build a working therapeutic relationship with each family member; 3) collect information about how the family currently functions including both strengths and challenges; and 4) to establish goals and objectives of the therapy. In Stage 2, the goals are to 1) help the family to better understand what it thinks about itself through circular and open-ended questions that allow family members to challenge current beliefs and assumptions and potentially open new possibilities for change. In Stage 3 of SyFT, the therapist promotes further consideration, refinement, and the addition of new information related to the themes identified in Stage 2. Thus, the content and process of these sessions are often considerably different from those in Stage 2. For example, in Stage 3 it is common for the therapist to focus on encouraging change, reframing ideas, and promoting consideration of new explanations for how the family organizes itself and solves problems. SyFT concludes by asking the family to review their learning process during therapy while asking them to consider how what they have learned could help avoid future difficulties and plan for any anticipated future therapeutic needs.

Adolescent-Focused Therapy

Adolescent-focused therapy (AFT) is a manualized, psychodynamic approach based in self psychology. The therapeutic relationship is used to support the adolescent making necessary changes related to eating and self-care as well as to develop new strategies to cope with life's challenges, especially those associated with development during adolescence (Fitzpatrick et al. 2009). In an earlier iteration of AFT called *ego-oriented individual therapy* (EOIT), 37 female adolescents with AN were randomly assigned to receive family therapy or EOIT (Robin et al. 1999). While both treatments lead to similar improvements in eating-related psychopathology, family therapy was more effective in terms of weight restoration and return of menstruation. In a study of 121 adolescents with AN, FBT was compared with AFT. Although there were no statistical differences between the two treatments in terms of recovery (normalized weight and eating-related psychopathology), FBT showed statistically greater improvements in both BMI and eating-related psychopathology. At 6- and 12-month follow-up, recovery rates in FBT were about twice those in AFT. Nonetheless, adolescents who received AFT did improve considerably, and this approach is be considered a viable Level 2 (probably efficacious) empirically supported treatment.

AFT has three phases. In the first phase, the therapist collects information about the patient's family, developmental, and social history that is used to organize a case formulation to guide treatment. Another key aspect of phase one is the development of a therapeutic relationship that will, on the one hand, insist the adolescent eat enough and decrease exercise enough to begin to reverse starvation and, on the other hand, nurture and support the adolescent in taking up the physical, emotional, and developmental challenges that AN has been used to avoid. Usually these challenges fall into one of four major types:

1. *Regressive needs.* AN is used to avoid taking up the challenges of adolescent developmental tasks, thereby not taking up an adult role by increasing dependence on parents and family, avoiding exploring intimate and sexual relationships, and not asserting more independence from parents. Treatment focuses on encouraging taking up normal adolescent challenges and supporting the adolescent during this process.

2. *Anger/control issues.* AN is used as an indirect expression of anger toward parents or other family members and/or an attempt to exert control over others. Treatment focuses on fostering health and direct expression of conflict and anger and promoting more effective communication of these feelings.

3. *A depressive stance.* AN is used to manage feelings of helplessness and depression by using dieting and over-exercise as a strategy to avoid these feelings, thereby engendering a false sense of control. In addition, managing eating and weight issues may offer a false sense of achievement. Treatment also encourages facing strong feelings such as anger, depression, and helping the patient learn to tolerate them.

4. *Deficits in self-esteem.* AN is used as a strategy to feel accomplished and increase self-worth through overvaluation of weight and appearance. In these cases, AN may be a form of pseudo identity that substitutes for a real sense of self. Treatment is focused on helping the adolescent discover what her true values, interests, and aspirations are to promote the development of a sense of self.

In the second phase of AFT, the aim is to continue an in-depth exploration of the main themes of the case formulation and to anticipate any problems with relapse. It is the goal of the third phase to terminate treatment. This requires special attention because of the intense and meaningful therapeutic relationship that undergirds success in AFT.

Throughout all phases of AFT, collateral sessions with the adolescent parents are scheduled. These tend to occur more frequently as therapy is beginning and decrease over time. The purpose of these parental collateral sessions is to provide parents an update on the progress their child is making in AFT and solicit their input and support for their adolescent's efforts at overcoming AN.

Cognitive-Behavioral Therapy

Cognitive-behavioral therapy (CBT) focuses on identifying and restructuring links among thoughts, feelings, and behaviors stemming from AN. While this approach is well established in bulimia nervosa and binge-eating disorder (Agras et al. 2000), it may be less effective in AN, likely because of the ego-syntonic nature of the illness and limited motivation for change (Fairburn et al. 2003). CBT was used in a large randomized controlled trial for adolescent AN that compared it to treatment as usual and specialized inpatient psychiatric treatment for AN and found no differences in outcome between the groups except that CBT was more cost effective than the other approaches (Gowers et al. 2007). CBT meets Level 4 criteria as an experimental treatment for adolescent AN. Enhanced CBT (CBT-E) has been compared with psychodynamic therapy in a large randomized controlled trial, but there were no differences in outcome between the groups (Zipfel et al. 2014).

CBT typically progresses over four stages. During the first stage CBT is focused on treatment engagement, including development of a shared formulation of the cognitive, behavioral, and emotional maintaining factors for AN, education about the problems of ongoing AN in terms of medical and psychiatric outcomes, and establishment of weekly weighing and dietary and activity self-monitoring. These self-monitoring records are used to help establish patterns that normalize regular eating, including consistency with eating three meals and two or three snacks daily. Thus, stage one is largely focused on making meaningful behavioral changes to support clinical improvement. The second stage of CBT is focused on helping the patient challenge distorted beliefs and cognitions that serve to underlie behavioral changes. The third stage is aimed at integrating these cognitive and behavioral changes over time and in the context of ongoing life stresses and challenges. The final stage of CBT for AN is focused on relapse prevention by focusing on potential future threats to the gains made in therapy and identifying strategies to anticipate and minimize the impact of such threats by developing plans to address them.

Psychotropic Medications

There are no medications that are approved by the U.S. Food and Drug Administration for treating AN. The use of psychotropic medications in this population should be generally limited to the treatment of comorbid conditions such as anxiety or mood disorders that clearly predate the development of disordered eating (McKnight and Park 2010). It is important to remember that malnutrition can lead to symptoms that are very similar to the neurovegetative symptoms of depression, as well as heightened anxiety. Renourishment is the most appropriate intervention in cases where mood and anxiety symptoms have arisen solely in the context of malnutrition. Appetite-stimulating medications are typically not effective in this population, because this is a disorder of overcontrol rather than one of low appetite (Crow et al. 2009; Holtkamp et al. 2005; Medicine 1995; Walsh et al. 2006).

Treatments Illustrated

Medical Hospitalization

Bobby is a 15-year-old male who presented for psychiatric evaluation on recommendation from his pediatrician. In the year since his previous sports physical, he had lost 15 pounds, and he attributed this weight loss to being "more concerned about health." Bobby was running cross country with the school's varsity team and had also taken an interest in nutrition since viewing a documentary on the obesity epidemic in health class last year. Since that time, he focused on decreasing his sugar intake, minimizing intake of processed foods, and increasing his consumption of fruits and vegetables. As his weight decreased, his running times improved, and his coaches were quite happy with his performance in meets.

Parents reported that his self-esteem appeared to improve as a result of feeling included in team activities.

Bobby's pediatrician was concerned, because Bobby had been at normal weight prior to this weight loss but was now underweight. He presented with a heart rate of 42 beats per minute at rest, and his heart rate and blood pressure changed significantly (more than 40 beats per minute, and his systolic blood pressure goes from 110 to 80 mmHg) when he moved from lying to standing. Bobby endorsed feeling less energetic and more easily fatigued with daily workouts. He also reported difficulty with sleep and reported anxiety when faced with eating foods he had previously enjoyed. For example, he described feeling anxious and panicked when celebrating his older brother's birthday, because he did not want to eat birthday cake and was nervous that family members would comment. Parents noted that they thought that Bobby's focus on health and improved nutrition was a "good thing" given that he historically liked to eat a lot of candy and salty snacks. They had heard from his coach that he was a very disciplined runner and were proud of his recent accomplishments. He also appeared to be doing very well academically and was happy with his network of friends. He had recently confided in his older brother that he liked one of the girls on the cross-country team but was noticing a decrease in sexual interest as well as cessation of wet dreams in recent months.

Given the concern about weight loss and bradycardia, Bobby's pediatrician recommended inpatient hospitalization. Bobby's parents were quite surprised by this, because he appeared to be healthy and active. Bobby's father, in particular, had a lot of questions about what is considered "normal" for an athlete but consented to hospital admission for fear that Bobby was in medical danger. The adolescent medicine service recommended that Bobby remain on strict medical bed rest given that his overnight heart rate was 37 beats per minute. All of his laboratory studies were within normal limits, with the exception of his testosterone levels, which were quite low for his age. He was placed on a 2,500 kcal/day meal plan to approximate his intake at home, and his caloric intake was increased by approximately 200 kcal/day. His electrolytes, including magnesium and phosphorus, remained within the normal range over the course of his hospitalization.

During the medical hospitalization Bobby met with the psychiatry team. He denied feeling that he was fat but did endorse worry about gaining weight were he to increase his intake. He also endorsed difficulty increasing his intake, despite the fact that he was being told that he needed to do so. He specifically worried about his running times and expressed concern that he would be "too heavy" if he ate all of the food that he was being given on the unit. He was diagnosed with anorexia nervosa of the restrictive type, but his parents were concerned about the label and needed extensive psychoeducation and discussion to come to terms with the diagnosis. His father, in particular, did not see how his son could possibly have an illness that he conceptualized as being a problem for "rich white girls." However, as they were able to see Bobby's response to renourishment, they gradually came to agree with the diagnosis.

Over the course of hospitalization, Bobby also complained of constipation, bloating, and postprandial abdominal pain, which improved over time. He also endorsed relief from warm packs after meals in addition to daily stool softener to regulate bowel movements. He initially said that he would do "whatever I need to get out of here and get back to running," but as his caloric requirements increased, he became very anxious and had a lot of difficulty eating. He also had trouble with bed rest, because he wanted to be able to go out for a run. He was caught doing pushups and situps in the bathroom and was found to be running in place in the middle of the night. This made it necessary for him to have staff with him at all times for support and redirection so that he did not act on his strong impulses to exercise.

Bobby's parents were present at the bedside most of the times and at least one of them participated in all meals and snacks. They met with the nursing staff before and after each meal to plan and to discuss their observations and over time came up with strategies to encourage Bobby to eat, even when he felt overwhelmed and physically uncomfortable. As they began to see his difficulty with restoring nutrition, they were more comfortable with the diagnosis but felt strongly that the psychiatrist on the unit work intensively to "change his mindset" about eating. They felt that Bobby would be able to recover easily if he just had the proper education about his body's needs. The psychiatrist met with Bobby on a daily basis to provide psychoeducation, explore his concerns, and to teach relaxation and coping strategies. Bobby stated that he understood why he needed to eat more but admitted that he continued to struggle to do so. The psychiatrist also met with the family to provide psychoeducation about anorexia nervosa, including externalizing the illness. They agreed that, in healthy moments, Bobby seemed to acknowledge and agree with the need for treatment. However, when faced with a large meal, he seemed to become easily overwhelmed and adamant that he did not need to eat.

After a 17-day admission, Bobby's vital signs had stabilized, and he had gained about 6 pounds. The adolescent medicine team felt that he was ready to return home. The family was in agreement with following up with a dietitian and the adolescent medicine team, as they agreed that it was important to monitor his health status and to optimize his nutrition in order to get back to running at an elite level. However, they were less interested in psychological treatment. They worried that needing to take time away from school and activities would make Bobby feel different from his friends, and they worried that this would have a negative impact on him. They also expressed concern that "dwelling too much on this" would be counterproductive. They desperately wanted Bobby to get back to school and back to cross-country as quickly as possible.

The pediatrician was able to work with the hospital team, including adolescent medicine, psychiatry, and the dietitian, to help Bobby's parents understand the need for ongoing psychiatric care. All team members were sure to support and reinforce mental health recommendations during the admission. Options for outpatient care were discussed at length with the family. They understood that FBT had the most evidence to support its use in adolescents, and they preferred keeping Bobby with them at home rather than sending him to a specialized eating disorder or residential program. They were motivated to be aggressive with treatment in hopes that it would allow speedy recovery from the illness and were in agreement with taking control of planning, purchasing, preparing, and plating all meals and snacks.

Residential Treatment for Persistent Anorexia Nervosa

Sally is a 23-year-old female who has been struggling with undiagnosed and untreated anorexia nervosa since the age of 16. She presented to a psychiatry clinic with concerns about anxiety and depression and was requesting medications to target these symptoms. However, her physician noted her low weight and screened for eating disorder symptoms. When it became clear that her signs and symptoms met criteria for anorexia nervosa, her psychiatrist discussed her options with her. She was encouraged to involve her family in treatment but did not believe that this was a viable option given that her parents were divorced and she had no relationship with her father. Her mother struggled with substance dependence and was not willing to take on the responsibility for renourishing her daughter because, as she told Sally, "It is too difficult to tolerate your distress." Sally was disappointed but accepted her family's limitations. She agreed that her symptoms of depression and anxiety were secondary to malnutrition, as she had never experienced them when she was adequately nourished. Sally's new psychiatrist recommended that she be medically evaluated urgently given the length of illness she had experienced.

Sally met with her internist, who found that her vital signs were normal. However, her BMI was 15, and she was experiencing ongoing urges to restrict her intake and to exercise compulsively. She denied any binge-eating or purging behavior. She acknowledged low mood, fatigue, and low energy but denied any suicidal ideation or self-injurious behavior. She also endorsed significant anxiety when attempting to eat but denied a history of premorbid anxiety symptoms.

Sally and her psychiatrist initially decided on a trial of CBT with a focus on increasing her intake and decreasing her activity. She was referred to a psychologist with eating disorder expertise and met with this clinician for five sessions. She attended all sessions and engaged appropriately in self-monitoring her behaviors. Despite her motivation to recover and sincere engagement in treatment, Sally experienced a 10-pound weight loss in this time. While she was not medically unstable, she no longer felt in control of her actions and acknowledged that she was unable to control her urges to overexercise and restrict intake.

Sally's therapist referred her to a local partial hospitalization program (PHP). She was able to take a few weeks off work to engage completely in the program. She found it helpful to have support at mealtimes but continued to struggle to take in enough to support the amount of activity that she was doing when she left the program for the day. She routinely engaged in running and exercise videos after hours. She found it difficult to control her behavior because she lived alone and was not able to count on her parents to help her moderate her activity and intake.

Her PHP made the recommendation that she think about residential treatment, and she was in agreement with making that change. She entered into residential treatment and was able to make progress with weight restoration and renourishment. Her mood and anxiety improved, and she felt that things were in a better place. She was following a meal plan, and her activity was monitored by the residential unit.

Sally was able to make adequate progress in the residential treatment center and was discharged home. She returned to work and was encouraged to reconnect to her outpatient team. Despite the significant work that she did in the residential setting, Sally struggled with this lower level of support. She found it relatively easy to decrease her intake at meals and even skip meals without the oversight provided by the residential setting. Within days, she was restricting her intake and overexercising. Her mother expressed concern about her behavior but was not willing to take on responsibility of helping Sally to change her behaviors.

Although her vital signs were stable, Sally continued to experience difficulty with her intake and was losing weight. A long-term friend and work colleague expressed concern and was willing to support Sally through this difficult time. She allowed Sally to move in with her, with the caveat that Sally would not be able to continue to live there if she was not involved in active treatment. Sally was able to reconnect with her outpatient therapist and was able to make progress with the structure and support of her friend in place. Sally was able to see that having her family involved would be ideal but could see that having accountability in any form would encourage her to take in enough to remain medically stable. Sally was able to make medical progress, remain in her job, and stay out of a higher level of care.

Family-Based Treatment for Anorexia Nervosa

Bobby, the 15-year-boy discussed earlier who had been hospitalized for medical instability for 17 days prior to starting FBT, was not enthusiastic about his parents being involved in treatment. He also did not see why his 18-year-old brother needed to attend.

The therapist in the first session of FBT endeavors to help the entire family understand the seriousness of AN and the impact the illness was having on the patient and the family as a whole. In FBT in the first phase of treatment, parents are asked to take control of all renourishment activities, much like nurses had done on the inpatient medical unit. Understandably, Bobby's parents were not confident in their abilities to refeed their son, because prior to his hospitalization he had successfully thwarted their efforts. However, the therapist reminded them that they had been successful in feeding their children up to this point, so they really had the necessary skills and knowledge if they could regain confidence in their approach. AN was externalized—that is, described as a disease, like cancer, that was threatening Bobby's life—and it was their job to make sure he received the treatment he needed, in this case, sufficient food to restore his weight. Bobby's parents felt guilty and responsible for potentially having caused AN to develop in their son, and this made them feel anxious about making any intervention for fear of making things worse. The therapist told them that the cause of AN is unknown and that there is no evidence that parents or family problems are specific causes of AN. The therapist also reminded Bobby's parents that without treatment, Bobby could again become medically unstable with potentially life-threatening cardiac irregularities. In addition, the therapist reminded the parents of the medical and psychological impacts of AN and starvation, including bone loss, hair loss, growth failure, and endocrine suppression. They were reminded that AN has the highest mortality risk of any psychiatric disorder due to cardiac arrest and suicide. By emphasizing the seriousness AN, the therapist sought to mobilize the parents to take immediate action to refeed their son.

The second session of FBT involves the parents bringing a family meal to the therapist's office so the therapist can experience in vivo with the family their current efforts for helping their child eat as directed by the therapist at the end of session 1. Bobby's parents had discussed together what to bring. The meal consisted of a turkey sandwich without dressing or cheese; water; and a fruit cup. When asked how they decided on this meal, the parents said that this was a meal that they thought Bobby might eat. When pressed further about whether they thought if Bobby ate this meal it would lead to significant weight gain, they said that if he ate it they would be pleased as a starting point but acknowledged that he would need to eat much more if he were to truly make weight progress. The therapist asked how they would modify the meal to address this and both parents stated that adding mayonnaise and cheese to the sandwich and adding chips and a milkshake to the meal would definitely be more likely to lead to significant weight gain. The therapist complimented the parents on their knowledge about what they knew would help nutritionally but worried about why they did not actually bring that meal. The parents said that they were afraid that Bobby would not eat at all if they had brought such a meal. At this point the therapist asked what the parents would do if Bobby needed a medication to treat a medical illness—would they give him half the dose he needed if he refused to take the whole dose? The parents said they would make him take the whole dose. The therapist reminded them that in the case of AN, food is medicine and that he needs his entire dose. Bobby sat listening to this discussion while tearing off the crust of the bread on his sandwich. He had not eaten anything but had finished the bottle of water. The therapist asked Bobby if he had eaten all he planned to eat. Bobby replied that he had and he would eat more later. The therapist turned to the parents and asked if they thought Bobby had eaten enough to gain weight. They agreed he had not. The therapist then asked the parents to try to help Bobby eat more. They began by asking him to eat. He refused. The therapist reminded the parents that AN is an illness and that it makes it very difficult for Bobby to agree to eat when they ask. Instead, the therapist asked the parents to tell Bobby that he must eat. The parents struggled at first to do this and each parent was saying something different to Bobby. The therapist reminded the parents that having clear expectations and agreements about what they expect of their children is something they have always done for other things, and they needed to find a way to do this now. The therapist encouraged the parents to agree on exactly what they wanted Bobby to eat and to sit on either side of him telling him in the same words together what they expected. Bobby tried to push his chair away, but the parents were able to keep him at the table. Bobby started to cry but eventually ate several bites of the sandwich. The therapist complimented the parents on how well they worked together and their success at helping Bobby eat. The therapist also consoled Bobby by saying it was very hard for Bobby to fight AN and that by listening to his parents and doing as they had asked he was showing the healthy part of him was still able to challenge AN. Bobby did not reply directly to this and continued to weep.

Over the rest of the first phase of FBT, the parents were able to discuss successes and challenges in renourishing Bobby each week. They discussed ways that they would typically handle challenging behavior and considered a range of possible strategies from the knowledgeable therapy that included approaches other families had successfully utilized to support their children in similar situations. However, the decision about which approaches to try was left completely up to the parents.

Bobby was weighed at the beginning of each session, and the weight set the tone for the meeting. After meeting independently with the therapist at the beginning of each session, Bobby was joined by the entire family to review how things were going that week. In the beginning, Bobby was quite irritable and annoyed that his brother needed to take time away from homework and after-school activities in order to attend sessions. He experienced a few weeks of attempting to refuse to eat and had many anger outbursts, but he continued to gain weight and his vital signs improved. He never reached a point of being a danger to himself or others.

Because of anger outbursts, his parents asked whether psychotropic medications could be helpful but ultimately agreed that it was important to see whether things improved with sustained nutrition and behavioral change. In a poignant moment, Bobby's brother expressed his worry for him, and this allowed the family to come together and find ways that the brothers could spend time together in a supportive manner. The parents struggled initially with taking control of meals and snacks because they valued independence and had encouraged their sons to take on increased autonomy. However, they were able to do so regularly once they saw that weight progression and improvement in vital signs seemed to be linked to how well Bobby ate that week.

Over time, Bobby was able to restore all of the weight that he had lost, and his vital signs were consistently stable. During the second phase of FBT, his parents were able to find ways to gradually allow him to take on more responsibility with meals and snacks, and over time, he was able to get to a point where he was plating his own meals with parent oversight to make sure that he was getting in enough nutrition. Despite his anxiety about weight gain and frustration with the process, Bobby was very motivated by getting healthy enough to return to training and being able to safely return to cross-country team activities. During the third phase of FBT, his parents allowed him to go back to running with his team, with the caveat that he would be forced to sit out practice if his weight was down that week. Over time, he was able to maintain his weight, return to sports, and had a successful academic career.

Adolescent-Focused Treatment for Anorexia Nervosa

Sonya is a 13-year-old female with an 8-month history of intentional weight loss by restricting her intake of all food, but particularly foods she thinks are fatty or high in protein. She is the only child of a single mother from Vietnam. Sonya is an excellent student but has no friends at her suburban high school. When beginning treatment with Sonya, the therapist found her to be a superficially friendly girl who seemed somewhat younger than 13. Sonya appeared to understand that her weight loss is potentially medically concerning, but she was not worried herself. She said that she likes how she feels when she does not eat. She noted that when she does not eat, she feels calmer and does not worry so much about her mother or her school work. Sonya reported that her mother must work a lot to afford to live in this expensive area and that her mother is often too tired to talk to her when she returns from work in the late evening. Sonya said she wanted to do well in school but that sometimes it was hard, and she worried about how she would do on tests. She studied very late into the night. She thought her mother expected her to always get A's. Sonya has had few other activities and interests beside school work and now her diet.

In reviewing this information, the therapist developed a formulation that AN is serving Sonya by being a source of self-esteem and identity that helps to fill in her otherwise empty and limited social and familial environment. The therapist was able to develop a therapeutic relationship with Sonya fairly easily, in part because Sonya was so needy for attention. The therapist insisted that for them to work together, Sonya must begin to eat more and healthier foods with fat and protein in them. Sonya said she would try to do so, and at the beginning of each session the therapist weighed her and praised her if she had gained weight and expressed worries and concern if she had not.

Because Sonya had few interests outside of school work and dieting, the therapist was initially challenged to find ways to support exploring other avenues for Sonya to use to develop her sense of self and to explore adolescence. However, one interest Sonya mentioned was Asian boy bands. The therapist asked her to bring a recording of one of the groups she likes, and the two of them watched a video together. The therapist encouraged Sonya to discuss the music, what she liked or did not like, the appearance of the boys in the band, who she finds attractive and who not so much. Developing rapport through these exchanges, the therapist encouraged Sonya to explore her interest in developing peer relationships. As treatment progressed, the therapist asked Sonya to consider joining an after-school club or activity. She chose table tennis, because there were other Asian kids who were very active in that club. At first, she was too shy to play and just watched the others, but over time, with continued support from the therapist, she began to play as well.

The therapist held collateral sessions with Sonya's mother. She explained the treatment approach and how she would be trying to support Sonya gaining weight. She encouraged Sonya's mother to make sure there were adequate supplies of nourishing foods in the house and to ask Sonya for suggestions for new things she might be willing to try. In addition, the therapist emphasized how lonely Sonya was and suggested that although the mother had to work late, if she could find one or two evenings to set aside for Sonya that it would likely be helpful to both of them. Sonya's mother agreed with these suggestions and was able to follow through most of the time with them.

Sonya's weight steadily improved over the first 6 months of treatment, though weight progress was slower than the therapist had initially hoped. However, as Sonya began to have more social activities at school and outings with her mother on one or two evenings a week, she was able to eat more and gained weight more rapidly during the second half of treatment.

After about a year of treatment, Sonya was fully weight restored and no longer used undereating as strategy to cope with loneliness and feelings of emptiness. Instead, Sonya was now engaged in the early stages of adolescence with a few friends and a first crush on a boy from the table tennis club. The therapist discussed the progress that Sonya had made and began to plan for termination. At first Sonya was upset by the prospect of ending therapy, because she had developed a deep trust and affection for her therapist, but she also recognized that she was ready to try to move on with her life without the therapist. The therapist encouraged these thoughts and also suggested that she could contact the therapist at any time to update her on how she was doing and that the therapist would be available in the future if the need should arise.

Common Outcomes and Complications

- The length and course of AN are variable and are dependent on factors such as age at onset, length of illness prior to treatment, access to appropriate treatment, and severity of illness. Some recover quickly with rapid renourishment and aggressive, subspecialty treatment provided by experts in evidence-based treatments. Young patients whose illness is identified and treated quickly have the best prognosis.

- Others may experience a waxing and waning course of symptoms and may have periods of time when they are doing well alternating with episodes of acute deterioration.

- About 5% of individuals with AN are at risk of dying from complications of the illness. Death is often related to the medical complications of malnutrition, including cardiac dysrhythmia. However, a substantial number of deaths in patients with anorexia nervosa are due to suicide.

- While individuals with AN tend to be ambitious and hard-working, there is significant variability in the functional status of patients with active illness. Some are able to remain enrolled in school or work without difficulty, whereas others may need to take a leave of absence for treatment. Some are quite impaired and may be chronically disabled as a result of the illness.

Resources and Further Reading

Online Resources

Academy for Eating Disorders: www.aedweb.org
    Medical Care Standards Guide
American Academy of Child and Adolescent Psychiatry:
    www.aacap.org
    Facts for Families
    Practice Parameters
American Academy of Pediatrics: www.aap.org
    Policy Statement
American Psychiatric Association: www.psychiatry.org
    Clinical Practice Guidelines
National Eating Disorders Association:
    www.nationaleatingdisorders.org
Society for Adolescent Health and Medicine:
    www.adolescenthealth.org
    Position Statement

Training Resources

Cognitive-behavioral therapy: https://www.octc.co.uk/training
Family-based treatment: train2treat4ed.com

Lock J, LeGrange D: Treatment Manual for Anorexia Nervosa: A
    Family-Based Approach, 2nd Edition. New York, Guilford, 2013
Fairburn CG: Cognitive Behavior Therapy and Eating Disorders.
    New York, Guilford, 2008

Further Reading

Collins L, Bulik C: Eating With Your Anorexic: A Mother's Memoir.
    Warrenton, VA, Biscotti Press, 2014
LeGrange D, Lock J: Eating Disorders in Children and Adolescents:
    A Clinical Handbook. New York, Guilford, 2011
Lock J, LeGrange D: Help Your Teenager Beat an Eating Disorder,
    2nd Edition. New York, Guilford, 2015
Mehler P, Andersen A: Eating Disorders: A Guide to Medical Care
    and Complications, 2nd Edition. Baltimore, MD, Johns Hopkins
    University Press, 2010
Musby E: Anorexia and Other Eating Disorders: How to Help Your
    Child Eat Well and Be Well. APRICA, 2014
Schaefer J: Life Without Ed: How One Woman Declared Indepen-
    dence From Her Eating Disorder, and How You Can Too, 2nd Edi-
    tion. New York, McGraw-Hill, 2014
Schaefer J: Goodbye, Ed, Hello Me: Recover From Your Eating Disor-
    der and Fall in Love With Life. New York, McGraw-Hill, 2009

Treasure J, Smith G, Crane A: Skills-Based Learning for Caring for a
Loved One With an Eating Disorder: The New Maudsley
Method. East Sussex, UK, Routledge, 2007

References

Agras WS, Walsh T, Fairburn CG, et al: A multicenter comparison of
cognitive-behavioral therapy and interpersonal psychotherapy for
bulimia nervosa. Arch Gen Psychiatry 57(5):459–466, 2000 10807486

Agras WS, Lock J, Brandt H, et al: Comparison of 2 family therapies
for adolescent anorexia nervosa: a randomized parallel trial.
JAMA Psychiatry 71(11):1279–1286, 2014 25250660

American Psychiatric Association: Diagnostic and Statistical Manual
of Mental Disorders, 5th Edition. Arlington, VA, American Psychiatric Association, 2013

Anderluh MB, Tchanturia K, Rabe-Hesketh S, et al: Childhood obsessive-compulsive personality traits in adult women with eating
disorders: defining a broader eating disorder phenotype. Am J
Psychiatry 160(2):242–247, 2003 12562569

Birmingham CL, Su J, Hlynsky JA, et al: The mortality rate from anorexia nervosa. Int J Eat Disord 38(2):143–146, 2005 16134111

Brewerton TD, Costin C: Long-term outcome of residential treatment
for anorexia nervosa and bulimia nervosa. Eat Disord 19(2):132–
144, 2011a 21360364

Brewerton TD, Costin C: Treatment results of anorexia nervosa and
bulimia nervosa in a residential treatment program. Eat Disord
19(2):117–131, 2011b 21360363

Crow SJ, Mitchell JE, Roerig JD, et al: What potential role is there for
medication treatment in anorexia nervosa? Int J Eat Disord
42(1):1–8, 2009 18683884

Fairburn CG, Cooper Z, Shafran R: Cognitive behaviour therapy for
eating disorders: a "transdiagnostic" theory and treatment. Behav Res Ther 41(5):509–528, 2003 12711261

Fairburn CG, Cooper Z, Shafran R: Enhanced cognitive behavioral
therapy for eating disorders ("CBT-E"): an overview, in Cognitive
Behavioral Therapy and Eating Disorders. Edited by Fairburn
CG. New York, Guilford, 2008, pp 23–34

Fitzpatrick KK, Moye A, Rienecke R, et al: Adolescent focused therapy for adolescents with anorexia nervosa. J Contemp Psychother
40(1):31–39, 2009

Forsberg S, Lock J: Family based treatment of child and adolescent
eating disorders. Child Adolesc Psychiatr Clin N Am 24(3):617–
629, 2015 26092743

Godart N, Berthoz S, Curt F, et al: A randomized controlled trial of
adjunctive family therapy and treatment as usual following inpatient treatment for anorexia nervosa adolescents. PLoS One
7(1):e28249, 2012 22238574

Golden NH, Attia E: Psychopharmacology of eating disorders in children and adolescents. Pediatr Clin North Am 58(1):121–138, xi, 2011 21281852

Golden NH, Katzman DK, Sawyer SM, et al: Update on the medical management of eating disorders in adolescents. J Adolesc Health 56(4):370–375, 2015 25659201

Gowers SG, Clark A, Roberts C, et al: Clinical effectiveness of treatments for anorexia nervosa in adolescents: randomised controlled trial. Br J Psychiatry 191(5):427–435, 2007 17978323

Hatmaker G: Boys with eating disorders. J Sch Nurs 21(6):329–332, 2005 16419341

Herpertz-Dahlmann B, Schwarte R, Krei M, et al: Day-patient treatment after short inpatient care versus continued inpatient treatment in adolescents with anorexia nervosa (ANDI): a multicentre, randomised, open-label, non-inferiority trial. Lancet 383(9924):1222–1229, 2014 24439238

Holtkamp K, Konrad K, Kaiser N, et al: A retrospective study of SSRI treatment in adolescent anorexia nervosa: insufficient evidence for efficacy. J Psychiatr Res 39(3):303–310, 2005 15725429

Jáuregui-Garrido B, Jáuregui-Lobera I: Sudden death in eating disorders. Vasc Health Risk Manag 8:91–98, 2012 22393299

Jones DV: Body image and the appearance culture among adolescent girls and boys: an examination of friend conversations, peer criticism, appearance magazines, and the internalization of appearance ideals. J Adolesc Res 19(3):323–339, 2004

Lock J: Trying to fit square pegs in round holes: eating disorders in males. J Adolesc Health 44(2):99–100, 2008 19167655

Lock J: An update on evidence-based psychosocial treatments for eating disorders in children and adolescents. J Clin Child Adolesc Psychol 44(5):707–721, 2015 25580937

Lock J, Le Grange D: Treatment Manual for Anorexia Nervosa: A Family Based Approach. New York, Guilford, 2013

Lock J, Couturier J, Agras WS: Comparison of long-term outcomes in adolescents with anorexia nervosa treated with family therapy. J Am Acad Child Adolesc Psychiatry 45(6):666–672, 2006 16721316

Lock J, Le Grange D, Agras WS, et al: Randomized clinical trial comparing family based treatment with adolescent-focused individual therapy for adolescents with anorexia nervosa. Arch Gen Psychiatry 67(10):1025–1032, 2010 20921118

Lock J, La Via MC, American Academy of Child and Adolescent Psychiatry Committee on Quality Issues: Practice parameter for the assessment and treatment of children and adolescents with eating disorders. J Am Acad Child Adolesc Psychiatry 54(5):412–425, 2015 25901778

McKnight RF, Park RJ: Atypical antipsychotics and anorexia nervosa: a review. Eur Eat Disord Rev 18(1):10–21, 2010 20054875

Medicine S: A position statement of the Society for Adolescent Medicine. J Adolesc Health 16(5):413, 1995 7662693

Mehler PS, Brown C: Anorexia nervosa—medical complications. J Eat Disord 3:11, 2015 25834735

Pote H, Stratton P, Cottrell D, et al: Systemic family therapy can be manualized: research process and findings. J Fam Therapy 25(3):236–262, 2003

Robin AL, Siegel PT, Moye AW, et al: A controlled comparison of family versus individual therapy for adolescents with anorexia nervosa. J Am Acad Child Adolesc Psychiatry 38(12):1482–1489, 1999 10596247

Skipper A: Refeeding syndrome or refeeding hypophosphatemia: a systematic review of cases. Nutr Clin Pract 27(1):34–40, 2012 22307490

Smink FRE, van Hoeken D, Oldehinkel AJ, et al: Prevalence and severity of DSM-5 eating disorders in a community cohort of adolescents. Int J Eat Disord 47(6):610–619, 2014 24903034

Walsh BT, Kaplan AS, Attia E, et al: Fluoxetine after weight restoration in anorexia nervosa: a randomized controlled trial. JAMA 295(22):2605–2612, 2006 16772623

Yager JDM: Practice Guideline for the Treatment of Patients with Eating Disorders, 3rd Edition. Washington, DC, American Psychiatric Association, 2006

Zipfel S, Wild B, Gross G, et al: Focal psychodynamic therapy, cognitive behaviour therapy, and optimised treatment as usual in outpatients with anorexia nervosa (ANTOP study): randomised controlled trial. Lancet 383(9912):127–137, 2014 24131861

Chapter 3

Bulimia Nervosa

Athena Robinson, Ph.D.

Nina Kirz, M.D.

Introduction

Bulimia nervosa (BN), "an ominous variant of anorexia nervosa," was first described a full century after anorexia nervosa by Gerald Russell in 1979. Subsequently, research and observation on all facets of the illness surged, and therefore its name, presentation, and sequelae rapidly garnered attention and infamy as a significant illness. Nowadays it is colloquially referred to among not only healthcare providers but also laypersons.

BN is known primarily for its two core features: recurrent objective binge episodes followed by purposeful compensatory behavior. The binge eating is characterized by the "out of control" consumption of a large amount of food within a short period of time. Compensatory behaviors are any behavior employed by the individual in order to "rid" himself or herself of the food (i.e., calories, fat) and often the sensation of physical distention/bloat incurred from the binge-eating episode. The most well-known and commonly referred to compensatory behavior is self-induced vomiting, although the range of diagnostic qualifying methods can include laxative or diuretic abuse, fasting (i.e., going up to 8 consecutive hours without eating), and excessive exercise.

BN has profound psychological (including social and emotional) and physical consequences for the individuals affected. As with any of the eating disorders, early detection and triage to efficacious interventions is highly recommended.

This chapter provides a practical and fundamental guide to understanding and treating BN. We review diagnostic criteria, diagnostic rule outs, risks and epidemiology, and medical and psychiatric comorbidities as well as provide an overview of efficacious treatments and case examples.

Key Diagnostic Checklist

❏ Recurrent episodes of both binge eating and inappropriate compensatory behaviors. Objective binge episodes are eating episodes in which both of the following apply:

   1. An unambiguously large amount of food is eaten within a discrete period of time (i.e., within a 2-hour period). "Unambiguously large" may be thought of a quantity that can be divided into two meals or that which would not be considered normative given the context and circumstances. It is not based on total caloric intake, because some objective binge episodes may include low-calorie, dense foods such as fruits or vegetables. Examples of unambiguously large episodes may include four bagels with spread or one box of cereal or six bananas (for additional examples, see the appendix of the Eating Disorder Examination [EDE; Fairburn and Cooper 1993]).

   2. A sense of loss of control over the eating episode. *Loss of control* refers to the individual's sense that they cannot stop eating once they have begun or that they cannot stop eating until all of the food is gone.

❏ Compensatory behaviors are behaviors that are employed in order to purposefully compensate (i.e., get rid of, negate, decrease the impact of) calories or fat ingested during a binge-eating episode. Compensatory behaviors may include any of the following (multiple may apply): self-induced vomiting, laxative misuse, fasting (i.e., going 6 or more hours without eating), or excessive exercise.

   • Both the binge eating and inappropriate compensatory behavior occur on average at least once per week over the course of 3 months.

   • Self-evaluation is unduly influenced by body shape and weight.

❏ The symptoms do not occur exclusively within an episode of anorexia nervosa.

Some individuals will have multiple cycles of binge eating and purging immediately following one another, whereas others will have a single cycle. An example of multiple cycles is binge eat, purge, immediately return to binge eating (as the first purge "made space" for the immediate return to binge eating), purge, and repeat. An example of a single cycle is binge eat, purge, and then end for that segment of time. Clinicians are encouraged to inquire about the composition of the individual's episodes and whether or not he or she experiences single or multiple cycles.

Although the method to induce vomiting is irrelevant in the diagnostic assignment of BN, clinicians are encouraged to assess the method(s) used in order to better understand the severity and/or duration of illness.

- To self-induce vomit, most individuals with BN use their fingers to prompt their gag reflex and vomit. Over time however, some individuals report that they no longer need to use their fingers in order to vomit and that the act of bending over alone will elicit the vomiting response.
- Some individuals with BN use an object (i.e., toothbrush or spoon) to prompt the gag reflux and vomiting behavior. It is always important to assess for esophageal damage and rupture in BN, but particularly in cases when the individual is using a foreign object to facilitate purging.

Clinicians beginning to work with BN patients often ask, "What exactly is *excessive* exercise"? There is no exact quantity defined by DSM-5 that fits the construct of *excessive*, as the concept typically relates more to the quality of the exercise rather than the quantity alone per se. However, clinicians have often used the following to facilitate their assessment and determination of the excessive exercise behavior. (*Note:* Special considerations may apply for athletes at the collegiate, elite, and/or Olympic levels.)

- Is the exercise "driven and compelled"? In other words, will the individual feel notably guilty if it is not completed, as though he or she has done something wrong?
- Does the timing of the exercise indicate its compensatory nature? Is it completed immediately after the binge-eating episode?
- What does the individual report as the purpose of the exercise? Most individuals with BN will endorse that the exercise is used specifically to rid oneself of the "damage done" via the binge-eating episode.

- Is the exercise completed while injured or physically ill? Positive endorsement supports an excessive quality to the exercise.

Consultation with colleagues on what may or may not qualify as excessive exercise is recommended as needed.

Having a thorough understanding of a patient's physical health profile will augment clinicians' ability to comprehensively assess the case and tailor interventions accordingly. Indeed, medical assessment in BN is critical because it can identify health problems related to the BN. In addition, medical assessment can highlight the severity of physical ramifications caused by the BN. For example, some individuals with BN report conditions (acid reflux, gastroparesis) that impact the schedule of eating and the quantity consumed. Likewise, allergies, inflammatory bowel disease, and Crohn's or celiac disease may influence food selection and report of subsequent gastrointestinal discomfort. Weight loss, gain, or fluctuation due to medical conditions such as hypo- or hyperthyroidism, cancer, and diabetes must also be ruled out.

BN is associated with a striking number of psychiatric comorbidities. About 95% of individuals with BN may have a comorbid psychiatric condition (Hudson et al. 2008). Mood disorders are the most common comorbidities in eating disorders in general. Anxiety disorders are also common. Studies consistently show that substance use and impulse-control disorders are more frequently seen in BN than in AN samples (Bulik et al. 2004; Hudson et al. 2008).

Diagnostic Rule Outs

- *Other eating disorders*
  - If the symptoms of BN occur within the context of anorexia nervosa, then the diagnosis of anorexia nervosa binge/purge subtype is more appropriate than BN.
  - The per-week frequency of binge and purge episodes endorsed will distinguish BN from other specified feeding and eating disorder (OSFED)—BN of low frequency. Frequency will also indicate the severity label to be added to the diagnosis: mild (1–3), moderate (4–7), or severe (8–13).

- If there are no objective binge-eating episodes, a diagnosis of OSFED—purging disorder should be considered.

- *Disorders that involve impulsivity, such as impulse-control disorder and borderline personality disorder.* Both diagnoses involve symptoms of behavioral and emotional dysregulation and disturbances in self-control. Individuals with BN may indeed act impulsively in regard to eating and other arenas, but in order for the diagnosis to be assigned, their symptoms must meet full criteria for BN. Impulse-control disorder and borderline personality disorder would not be assigned if the impulsivity was only circumscribed to eating and purging behavior.

- *Comorbid gastrointestinal pathology.* Such pathology may mimic purging side effects (e.g., celiac sprue, celiac disease, Crohn's disease, food allergy–induced diarrhea, and weight loss) or limit an individual's ability to eat and/or digest meal portions expected for the age and/or sex (e.g., gastroparesis) and should be assessed and ruled out as needed.

Epidemiology and Risk Factors

Epidemiology

- The 12-month prevalence of BN is 1%–1.5% among adolescent and young adult women (American Psychiatric Association 2013).
- Lifetime prevalence has been estimated to be 0.5% and 1.3% among boys and girls, respectively (Swanson et al. 2011).
- Data garnered from treatment-seeking samples indicate that the gender ratio is approximately 3:1 for women to men.
- Peak age at onset tends to be late adolescence to young adulthood.
- While data show that binge eating is the most commonly occurring form of disordered eating among minorities, data are mixed as to whether rates of BN specifically differ among racial and ethnic groups. Nonetheless, BN affects a wide range of racial and ethnic groups.
- The mortality rate of BN is less than that of anorexia nervosa; however, it is still elevated in comparison to the rate in the general population.

- Suicide risk and rates of suicide attempts and completed suicide are elevated in BN compared with the general population and occur in 25%–35% of those with the illness.
- Longer-term follow-up studies suggest that approximately 50% of individuals achieve and sustain recovery.

Risk Factors

- *Dieting.* Studies suggest that dieting may precede onset of binge eating and bulimic and eating pathology.
- *Tendency toward overeating.* Dieting may be a proxy for a tendency toward overeating.
- *Fasting.* Fasting behavior appears to increase the reward value of food increasing the risk for binge eating.
- *Stress and negative mood.* These are frequent precipitants of binge eating (Polivy and Herman 1993).
- *High reward of eating.* Individuals with BN rate food pictures more arousing and endorse higher desires to eat, even when sated, compared with those who do not binge eat (Karhunen et al. 1997).
- *Impulsivity.* Individuals with BN demonstrate greater impulsivity compared with those without disordered eating (Guerrieri et al. 2007; Loxton and Dawe 2007); impulsivity includes behaviors such as self-mutilation, suicidal ideation, and heavy substance use (Penas-Lledó and Waller 2001; Pidcock et al. 2000; Vervaet et al. 2003).

Common Comorbidities

Medical

- *Cardiovascular.* Cardiac arrhythmias (abnormal heart rate), orthostatic blood pressure (drop in blood pressure upon standing), bradycardia (low pulse rate), syncope (fainting)

- *Gastrointestinal.* Parotid gland (or other salivary gland) enlargement, delayed gastric emptying, constipation, bloating, gastroparesis, esophageal damage from repetitive stomach acid exposure (tears, bleeding, tissue damage, ulcers)

- *Dental.* Enamel erosion and potential loss of teeth

- *Metabolic/Endocrine.* Electrolyte imbalance (i.e., decrease in potassium), vitamin deficiencies, decreases in growth hormones, pubertal delay, irregular menses, alkalosis (low pH from loss of stomach acid as detected in urine), edema (sodium retention)

- *Skeletal.* Osteopenia or osteoporosis (low bone density)

- *Dermatological.* Russell's sign (abrasions on the back of the hands caused by using one's own fingers to induce vomiting)

Psychiatric Comorbidities

- *Mood.* Depressive disorders

- *Obsessive-compulsive and related.* Obsessive-compulsive disorder

- *Trauma- and stress-related.* Posttraumatic stress disorder

- *Substance.* Substance use disorder, substance dependence, history of substance use disorder or dependence

- *Impulse control.* Pathological spending, gambling, internet use behaviors, kleptomania

- *Personality.* Cluster B, borderline personality disorder

Clinical Presentations

Case 1: Lindsey

Lindsey is a 19-year-old sophomore in university and a Division I athlete whose symptoms met criteria for BN. Based on her report, it appeared that Lindsey had previously had symptoms that met criteria for a major depressive episode in her sophomore year of high school. She reported onset of body image concerns around the time she was a junior in high school, prior to binge eating and purging. These behaviors began at a relatively low frequency (i.e., once every 2–3 months) in senior year of high school. Lindsey was highly devoted to her sport and wanted to improve her performance and believed losing weight was essential to accomplish her athletic goals. To accomplish this, when she arrived at college, she began restricting food. Specifically, she cut out carbohydrates and sweets. She lost weight, although her body mass index (BMI) remained within the low side of the normal range. It appeared at first that she was correct about losing weight improving her performance, but over time this approach proved to be unsupportable.

At the time of Lindsey's initial intake evaluation, she reported **basing her self-worth primarily on her weight and shape.** She also endorsed having **objective binge episodes approximately seven or eight times per week for about 1.5 years,** or since she was a freshman. A typical binge episode would include multiple bowls of cereal (at least one box worth) and perhaps four or five slices of bread with butter, eaten with an **experience of loss of control** that she could not stop the episode from proceeding once it began. Almost all of her binge food was obtained from the dormitory dining hall. After a binge, Lindsey would **purge via self-induced vomiting** in order to rid herself of the calories and fat she had ingested. Sometimes Lindsey would continue a binge after an initial vomiting episode, and the cycle could repeat up to two or three times in one afternoon or sitting. At times, Lindsey would **use the exercise from her sport in order to also compensate** for her binge episodes. Lindsey reported both "hating" and "needing" her BN. She hated it because of the overwhelming amount of time she spent engaged in the behaviors of binge and purging as well as her seemingly ceaseless obsessionality with her body weight and shape. She stated she needed this obsessional preoccupation because she believed it helped keep her weight in check and thus allowed her to excel in her sports performance. Lindsey's family was unaware of the eating disorder, and she was resolved to not inform them. She was, however, willing to work with a physician on campus who regularly monitored her vital signs to ensure that she was medically stable enough for outpatient psychotherapy. Lindsey's BMI was 20, and she was menstruating regularly.

Case 2: Dillon

A 29-year-old man, Dillon, came for help with BN that had begun more than 12 years earlier. He traced body image concerns back to his early adolescent years, but he had begun binge eating and purging via self-induced vomiting only in high school, just after the divorce of his parents. The frequency and intensity of his symptoms had waxed and waned over the years, but their persistence and recent spike after the end of a romantic relationship prompted him to seek treatment for the first time.

Dillon endorsed having **objective binge episodes approximately once or twice per week** on a consistent basis **for**

several consecutive years. His work setting provided three meals daily, plus an open kitchen for snacks between meals, readily accessible to all employees. Dillon shared that this readily available open access to food made it a daily challenge to manage his food intake. He said he ate breakfast and lunch at the office daily, and these were followed by binge episodes starting in the late afternoon just prior to leaving the office. Dillon said that typically a binge-eating episode would begin about half an hour prior to departing work, when he would make repetitive trips to the kitchen to obtain two or three snack-sized bags of pretzels or chips, a handfuls of M&Ms or chocolate chips, and a few granola bars. He would then leave the office but stop on the way home at a local convenience store and purchase one or two large bags of candy such as chocolate bars and caramels (approximately 0.5–1 lb each). Upon arriving home, he would consume all of the candy within approximately 30–60 minutes, **experiencing a sense of loss of control over the eating, and then purposefully compensate for the calories ingested via self-induced vomiting.**

Dillon reported being so exhausted from these binge-and-purge cycles that he would go immediately to sleep once the cycle ended. He also said that his body weight and shape remained of high importance to him—in particular, his body composition being more muscular and less fatty. He felt he was failing at his goals in this regard, and this reduced his self-esteem.

Case 3: Georgia

Georgia is a 16-year-old high school junior. Her parents called to inquire about and potentially establish treatment for her because they were worried she had an eating disorder. They thought she was **obsessed with her weight** because she was always commenting about being overweight, checking her outfits and figure in the mirror, and asking for reassurance regarding her appearance multiple times throughout the day. Georgia also shared with her mother that she had occasionally made herself throw up after eating "too much."

In the initial assessment session, it was discovered that Georgia was binge eating regularly. She reported having **binge episodes** in secret about **two or three times per week,** and these were followed by **self-induced vomiting** and sometimes **laxatives** in order to compensate for the food she ate during a binge-eating episode. Georgia shared an example of a binge episode as consisting of eating two full sleeves of graham crackers (two-thirds of the box; about 16 full-sized crackers total) as well as about four "low-fat" ice-cream sandwiches. She felt out of control of her eating during these binge episodes and felt she could not stop eating once they began until she had consumed as much as possible. She also said she had binge-eating episodes when her family was out of the house after school or after they had gone to sleep for the night. She shared that she was buying laxatives from the drug store down the street from the family's home.

Georgia's weight was within normal limits for her height and sex, and she was regularly menstruating. Georgia had two brothers: a younger brother in eighth grade and an older brother who was away at college. Georgia's parents were quite worried about her. They wanted her to stop binge eating and purging and develop more positive self-regard and body image. They feared this if these behaviors continued they would hinder her ability to enjoy and benefit from the remainder of high school. They also worried about the disordered eating behaviors impacting her readiness for and potential independence at college.

Evidence-Based Outpatient Psychosocial Treatments for Bulimia Nervosa

Adults

Cognitive-behavioral therapy (CBT) (Fairburn et al. 2008)—Level 1 (established treatment)

Interpersonal psychotherapy (IPT) (Agras et al. 2000)—Level 1 (established treatment)

Dialectical behavior therapy (DBT) (Safer et al. 2001)—Level 1 (possibly efficacious)

Children and Adolescents

Family-based treatment (FBT) (Le Grange et al. 2015)—Level 2 (possibly efficacious)

Cognitive-behavioral therapy (Fairburn et al. 2008)—Level 1 (possibly efficacious)

Treatment Settings

The usual format of outpatient treatment for BN is standard 50- to 60-minute psychotherapy sessions once per week. The treatments discussed in this chapter (i.e., DBT, IPT, CBT, FBT) can follow this model. Patient and provider decisions about appropriate level of care should consider the medical stability and psychiatric safety (i.e., to prevent self-harm or harm to others). Outpatient forms of treatment are for patients who are medically stable, whereas higher levels of care are for those who require additional daily medical or psychiatric monitoring. Higher levels of care include intensive outpatient programs (approximately 3–5 hours per day within the treatment facility; patients return home to their regular living environment at the end of each day); partial hospitalization programs (patients reside within their facilities, which offer more intensive medical monitoring, but are not full-time residents); residential treatment (patients reside 24 hours a day in the facility and require intensive monitoring and treatment); and hospitalization (which for BN should be brief and used only when indicated for medical safety and psychiatric safety). Other than for medical necessity and psychiatric safety, it remains unclear when and for whom higher levels of care are beneficial for BN.

Regardless of the specific higher level of care used, all higher-level-care treatment providers should liaise with outpatient treatment providers to effectively and efficiently collaborate care and facilitate the transition from one modality to the other. To determine the medical stability of an individual, physicians are encouraged to refer to resources for the proper medical management of eating disorders, such as those put forth by the Academy for Eating Disorders (2016) and Golden et al. (2015).

Treatments

Cognitive-Behavioral Therapy

Enhanced cognitive-behavioral therapy (CBT-E) has been documented as the leading choice for psychotherapeutic interventions for BN by the National Institute for Health and Care Excellence (2017). Their 2017 guidelines gave CBT for BN a grade of A for the treatment of BN in adults; the grade indicates strong empirical support provided by well-conducted randomized, clinical trials. Among adults with BN, CBT has demonstrated superior outcomes compared with antidepressant medication (Wilson 2010), psychoanalytic psychotherapy (Poulsen et al. 2014), and interpersonal psychotherapy (IPT) at posttreatment (Agras et al. 2000). While CBT is a first-line treatment and many patients sustain recovery over the longer term, a significant minority are still symptomatic at the end of treatment. Thus, CBT is considered an efficacious treatment for BN in adults (Level 1).

Two randomized clinical trials with CBT-E—a newer version of CBT for BN that includes additional treatment modules to address perfectionism, low self-esteem, and interpersonal difficulties—were conducted with adult patients who had bulimic symptoms but did not have anorexia nervosa (Fairburn et al. 2009, 2015). Both studies found that approximately 75% of participants who began treatment achieved abstinence from binge eating and purging after 20 sessions of CBT-E. Furthermore, abstinence was maintained for the most part at 1-year follow-up.

CBT has also been examined in adolescents. A randomized comparison of CBT and FBT found that although FBT for BN was superior to CBT at the end of treatment, there were no statistical differences in outcome at 12-month follow-up, suggesting that both approaches may be useful but that FBT for BN may work faster (Le Grange et al. 2015). For adolescents, CBT is considered a possibly efficacious treatment (Level 2).

CBT-E is an enhanced version of the original version of CBT that 1) expands on techniques originally described in CBT, 2) has been adapted to address all forms of eating disorder (not solely BN), and 3) delineates additional illness-maintaining mechanisms that may become therapeutic focus. CBT-E is a time-limited treatment (often delivered in 20 individual sessions) that targets factors maintaining the illness cycle in an iterative fashion. A typical formulation used within CBT-E first involves appreciating the role that overevaluation of shape and weight and their control play is pivotal in understanding a patient's repetitive, poignant, and centralized emphasis on shape and weight and the co-occurring strong urge to control them via strict dietary restriction. Dietary restriction and noncompensatory weight control behavior (i.e., food rules about what, how much, and/or when something should or should not be eaten) poise humans for hunger and/or rule violation (often described as feeling a loss of control) and subsequent binge eating. As patients with BN will report, binge eating is necessarily followed by attempts to compensate for the ramifications of the binge via compensatory behaviors, renewed vows to restrict eating again, and magnification of shape and weight concerns. Second, the diagram illustrates the major influence of events and mood on binge eating that exacerbates the binge eating and purging cycle. Third, the diagram not only highlights the theoretical underpinning of BN-maintaining factors but also simultaneously pinpoints intervention targets (i.e., dieting, overevaluation of shape and weight, responsiveness to events and mood).

CBT progresses in four stages. Stage 1 focuses on several factors that aim to engage the patient in the treatment, including collaborative generation of BN formulation and its maintaining factors, psychoeducation, and establishment of weekly weighing and regular eating. *Regular eating* refers to the intervention of establishing consistency with eating three meals and two to three snacks daily and limiting eating outside of these episodes. Stage 2 transitions the patient from stage 1 to stage 3 via review of (and editing as needed) the formulation, identification of barriers to change, and progress to date. Stage 3 represents the largest focus of treatment; its goals are to tackle factors maintaining the BN while in the last stage of treatment. Examples of factors that may be maintaining the illness include body image concerns and dietary restraint, as well as events, mood, and other eating behaviors. The emphasis of stage 4 is on maintaining gains and minimizing relapse risk.

CBT can also be provided in a guided self-help format. *Pure self-help* (PSH) treatments are those that do not involve the assistance of a professional at any level and are primarily self-educational in format (e.g., books, content delivery websites). *Guided self-help* (GSH) treatments are those that are typically based in a particular therapeutic model, provide didactics on theoretically congruent skills or techniques, and involve limited guidance from a healthcare professional. Both PSH and GSH treatments are included as first-line interventions within the stepped-care treatment recommendations provided by the National Institute for Health and Care Excellence (2017). There are several benefits to GSH models, including improvement of treatment access at a decreased cost. However, serious clinical presentations are likely to require more intensity of treatment than can be provided through PSH and GSH.

Overcoming Binge Eating (Fairburn 1995, 2013) is a self-help manual that can be used as either PSH or GSH. It is the most well-researched self-help manual in the treatment of binge-eating disorders, including BN. When used as GSH, it is typically referred to as CBT-GSH, given the manual's theoretical foundation in CBT. This manual is broken up into two parts. Part I provides fundamental psychoeducation on the nature, etiology, and epidemiology of binge eating. Part II outlines a six-step iterative program for working toward binge eating abstinence. This manual is foundational for those interested in learning more about the CBT-GSH approach to the treatment of BN.

A meta-analysis of PSH and GSH among adults with BN, binge-eating disorder (BED), and other specified eating disorder (formally eating disorder not otherwise specified in DSM-IV [American Psychiatric Association 1994]) concluded that although PSH and GSH yielded significant reductions in eating disorder symptoms, interpersonal functioning, and some comorbid psychiatric symptoms, these results were not significantly different from those obtained with other treatments, including therapist-delivered psychotherapy (Perkins et al. 2006). Another meta-analysis concluded that PSH and GSH for binge-eating disorders (including BN) yielded outcomes significantly better than wait-list control conditions and that GSH tends to be superior to PSH (Stefano et al. 2006). For adolescents with bulimic behaviors, a randomized controlled trial comparing GSH with family therapy found no difference between the two modalities at the end of treatment (Schmidt et al. 2007).

Interpersonal Psychotherapy

IPT is a time-limited treatment that strives to improve interpersonal functioning and thereby reduce psychiatric symptoms via the consistent and purposeful focus on the relationship between symptoms, core interpersonal problem areas, and the establishment of alternative strategies for coping with said problems. IPT has substantial empirical support for the treatment of BN and is recommended as an alternative treatment to CBT-BN among adults (Wilson et al. 2007). While evidence indicates that IPT and CBT have equivalent longer-term outcomes in the treatment of BN, previous trials demonstrated that IPT-BN had a slower response time for symptom improvement than did CBT-BN. Thus, recommendations for IPT-BN suggest clinicians inform patients of this potential delayed response time. Moderator analyses exploring populations for whom IPT treatment may work better found that IPT, as compared with CBT, may be particularly well suited for African American women, who had greater reductions in binge-eating frequency when treated with IPT instead of CBT (Chui et al. 2007). In addition, some moderator data show that IPT may be fitting for individuals who present with greater general psychopathology (Markowitz et al. 2006; Wilfley et al. 2008). Last, IPT may be considered for patients who express discomfort with certain core elements of CBT-BN (i.e., food diary) (Tanofsky-Kraff and Wilfley 2009). Like CBT, IPT would also be ranked as a Level 1 evidence-based therapy for the treatment of BN. IPT has not been investigated among adolescents with BN. However, IPT for depression has demonstrated efficacy in this population, and thus the application of IPT for BN among adolescents may warrant investigation.

IPT for BN typically includes 15–20 sessions over 4–5 months (although brief forms of IPT are also available) and can be delivered in individual or group format. Problems in current interpersonal function and relationships can be classified into one of four social domains: grief, role disputes, role transitions, and interpersonal deficits. Domains are selected based on the pattern of associated onset with the eating disorder symptoms. *Grief* is selected when the eating disorder symptom onset is associated with the death of a loved one, recent or past. *Role disputes* is selected when the symptom onset is associated given conflicts with a significant other (partner, child, parent, professor, supervisor) regarding differential expectations of the relationship. When symptoms are linked to difficulties associated with a life status transition (promotion, marriage, divorce, retirement, starting college), *role transitions* is selected. Last, *interpersonal deficits* is selected when longstanding chronic patterns of social isolation or unfulfilling relationships are evident.

There are three phases in IPT treatment. During the initial phase, the clinician assigns the sick role, conducts the interpersonal inventory in order to arrive at the social domain, and establishes the interpersonal formulation and treatment contract. Assignment of the sick role is thought to reinforce the utility of treatment to address the documented, known condition while simultaneously identifying the need for help on the patient's behalf. Rather than being condescending, the sick role assignment is thought to alleviate the patient from other potentially conflicting obligations so that he or she can fully focus on the task of recovery. The Interpersonal Inventory is a key component of this initial phase because it facilitates identification of the primary social domain. It is conducted within the first few sessions and focuses on collaboratively generating a detailed review of the patient's current and past close relationships (including the patterns, functioning, and expectations within said relationships), with purposeful reference to both onset and maintenance of eating disorder symptoms. The interpersonal formulation, yielded from the work of the Interpersonal Inventory and including the specific social domain(s) to be addressed in treatment, is then developed and discussed with the patient. The intermediate phase maintains focus on the reciprocal relationship between the identified domain and the eating disorder symptoms. Each social domain has a specific list of strategies that are encouraged for use within the intermediate phase (Table 3–1). Other IPT techniques include encouraging expression of feeling, using role-plays to help take different perspective on relationships, analyzing communication styles, and using hypothetical situations and questions to introduce new possibility ways of relating to others, as well as using a detailed collaborative review of interpersonal incidents that occur during treatment. The termination phase focuses on reviewing progress and planning ahead for work that can continue beyond the end of formal treatment.

Dialectical Behavior Therapy

Dialectical behavior therapy (DBT) for eating disorders was adapted from the original DBT for borderline personality disorder (Linehan 1993a, 1993b). DBT is a comprehensive treatment approach that teaches cognitive and behavior change principles and skills for change yet remains nested within a framework of dialectical philosophy and Zen-based acceptance strategies (i.e., mindfulness). While the preliminary work on DBT for eating disorders with binge eating as a core symptom is promising, results are mostly limited to case reports, uncontrolled series, and uncontrolled trials. However, one randomized controlled trial compared DBT for BN (DBT-BN) with a wait-list control among 29 adult women and found that the rate of abstinence from binge eating and purging at 20 weeks posttreatment was 28.6% for DBT versus 0% for the wait-list (Safer et al. 2001). These DBT abstinence rates are comparable to posttreatment abstinence rates from a multisite study of CBT for BN (CBT-BN) (Agras et al. 2000). Im-

that DBT has demonstrated efficacy for impulsive behaviors among this population, the potential application of DBT-BN among adolescents may warrant investigation.

DBT for BED/BN, based on the affect regulation model of binge eating, postulates that intense negative affect can precede binge eating and that binge eating is used as a maladaptive means to regulate those emotions. Behaviors are addressed through teaching of skills in core categories (mindfulness; emotion regulation; distress tolerance), with integration of behavioral chain analyses of problem eating behaviors. The DBT model for BN developed at Stanford University includes 20 weekly 50- to 60-minute individual therapy sessions and was originally developed for adult women ages 18–65 years (Safer et al. 2001). There are important similarities and differences between the original DBT for borderline personality disorder and the Stanford DBT-BN model (Table 3–2).

In DBT-BN, treatment orientation and commitment to stop binge eating and purging occur in session 1; introduction of dialectical abstinence in session 2; mindfulness skills in sessions 3–5; emotion regulation skills in sessions 6–12; distress tolerance skills in sessions 13–18; and skills review alongside relapse prevention in sessions 19–20. The mindfulness module is the first in the series because it sets the foundation for the remainder of the therapy and skill application. Teaching promotes the benefits of being present in the moment, without judgment, and with full attention toward one-mindful and effective participation. Emotion regulation skills focus on teaching the purpose of emotions and how to understand their presence and label them accurately. This module also teaches some core strategies for reducing emotional intensity when the individual wishes to do so. Distress tolerance skills teach how to survive a crisis moment without making the situation worse. They acknowledge that pain is a part of life and that effective distress tolerance can mitigate the risk of making a situation worse. For example, binge eating may exacerbate a situation because it does not solve the original prompting event plus it adds physical and emotional suffering that could have otherwise been avoided.

Diary cards and chain analyses are also regularly used. Diary cards are structured forms on which patients indicate the occurrences of the week and what skills that have been using. They are reviewed at the outset of the therapy session and facilitate identifying the agenda for that session. Behavioral chain analyses are a collaborative approach the therapist and

TABLE 3–2. Similarities and differences in DBT for BPD and BN

DBT for BPD	DBT for BN
Individual + group therapy	Individual therapy[a]
Consultation team	No consultation team
1-year treatment	20 weeks of treatment
Four skills training modules (mindfulness, emotion regulation, distress tolerance, and interpersonal effectiveness)	Three skills training modules (mindfulness, emotion regulation, and distress tolerance)
Diary card	Diary card
Behavioral chain analysis	Behavioral chain analysis

Note. BN=bulimia nervosa; BPD=borderline personality disorder; DBT = dialectical behavior therapy.
[a]Safer et al. (2001) report that the choice to use individual therapy format for DBT-BN was fueled by difficulties in recruiting sufficient numbers to host a group instead.

patient undertake together in session to enhance understanding and clarity around why a particular behavior (e.g., binge eating and purging) took place and what skills could have been used to facilitate overcoming the urge to binge and purge.

Family-Based Therapy for Bulimia Nervosa for Adolescents

Historically, the involvement of the family in their child's recovery from an eating disorder was discouraged. However, mounting evidence suggests that instead of removing parents from treatment, strategically incorporating the family into interventions can yield promising results. FBT for BN (FBT-BN) is currently the most well researched and supported family inclusive form of treatment for adolescent BN. Although FBT for BN does not have as substantial an evidence base as FBT for anorexia nervosa in adolescents does, it is supported by findings from three randomized controlled trials conducted to date. FBT-BN was demonstrated to be significantly superior in achieving binge-eating and purging abstinence compared to supportive psychotherapy (delivered individually) among 80 adolescents with BN or partial BN at both posttreatment and 6-month follow-up (Le Grange and Lock 2007).

As noted earlier, CBT and FBT were compared in a large randomized controlled trial for adolescents with BN, and those adolescents receiving FBT achieved higher rates of abstinence from binge eating and purging at the end of treatment, but this difference was no longer significant at 12-month follow up. Moreover, moderator analysis indicated that families with lower levels of familial conflict had better outcomes when treated with FBT-BN instead of CBT. Taken together, this evidence suggests that FBT-BN has been supported as a possibly efficacious treatment for adolescents and as a viable alternative treatment to CBT delivered individually.

FBT-BN empowers the parents and the adolescent to collaboratively disrupt and cease destructive patterns of binge eating, purging, restrictive eating, and other forms of weight control behavior. The therapist, expert in BN in adolescence and well-trained in FBT, serves as a consultant to the family and facilitates the symptom-focused nature of treatment. In other words, the therapist aims to be nondirective and instead becomes an educator and sounding board for the family as they navigate the treatment process. This therapeutic stance allows the parents an opportunity to take ownership of treatment decisions and their implementation at home. The therapist uses strategies such as externalization, which serves to purposefully separate the adolescent from his or her illness, thereby promoting parental intervention and decreasing adolescent resistance to such assistance. Parents are charged with establishing structure surrounding eating and facilitating cessation of purging and other weight-control behaviors. Siblings, in contrast, are encouraged to be supportive throughout treatment and are not involved with feeding and purging cessation–related tasks.

A major difference between FBT-BN and FBT for AN is the role the patient takes in treatment. In FBT for AN, the adolescent wants to keep her illness and cannot be counted on to help with the treatment process until later on in therapy. In contrast, most adolescents with BN are ashamed of their illness and feel like failures at dieting. Engaging the family to help the adolescent with BN is a way to overcome this shame. This is accomplished in part by asking the adolescent to participate actively from the start of FBT-BN by identifying for his or her parents what foods trigger binge eating, when binge eating is likely to occur; how purging is done, and when. By bringing these behaviors into the light, the family can work together to help the adolescent to overcome them.

Treatment spans three phases. Phase I goals are to reestablish healthy eating; phase II is directed at facilitating the adolescent's ability to independently eat on his or her own; and, last, phase III focuses on adolescent issues and termination. All family members (parents, adolescent, siblings) attend all therapy sessions. Each session starts with a brief (i.e., no more than 15 minutes) meeting between the adolescent and therapist only. This time is dedicated to weighing the adolescent and reviewing a binge-eating and purging log, as well as building and maintaining rapport between the therapist and patient.

The parents and siblings then join the session. Each session in phase I focuses on ongoing parental empowerment at facilitating healthy eating in their child, encouragement of parental alliance on the specific methodology used at home to establish regular eating, involvement of the adolescent as a collaborative member of the treatment process, and provision of information about the physical and mental health consequences of BN. Weight and the binge eating and purging log are also discussed with the family each week.

The second session is a family meal. For this session the therapist invites the family to bring a picnic meal to session as well as a "forbidden food" or a food avoided or eaten under great distress by the adolescent with BN. The purpose of the picnic session includes launching the process of parental involvement in therapy, giving the therapist an opportunity to observe familial interactional patterns during a meal, and creating an opportunity for parents to encourage the adolescent's consumption of a forbidden food and affording them an opportunity to support their child through their anxiety and fears about binge eating, gaining weight, and purging. The remainder of phase I consists of weekly consultations with the family on their attempts to support their son or daughter in eating without binge eating, prevention of purging, and experimentation with feared or avoided foods.

Phase III is embarked on after the adolescent's eating patterns return to normal and the BN symptoms are largely eliminated. This phase involves a gradual transition of the adolescent back into an age-appropriate role of independence in control over his or her healthy eating behaviors. The focus is on increased personal autonomy and reestablishment of the interpersonal relationship between the adolescent and his or her parents that is separate from eating- and food-related behaviors.

Pharmacotherapy

The use of pharmacotherapy for the treatment of eating disorders has potential for several reasons. Specifically, medications can target neurobiological abnormalities that may not be fully responsive to psychotherapeutic approaches, augment approaches for chronic forms of the illnesses, prove useful in addressing comorbid psychiatric conditions, or address weight and appetitive regulation systems to facilitate tractability of behavioral interventions.

Studies suggest that CBT alone yields improved outcomes when compared with medication alone (Agras et al. 1992; Goldbloom et al. 1997; Walsh et al. 1997), and adding medication to CBT shows a modest benefit compared with CBT alone (Agras et al. 1992; Walsh et al. 1997) Thus, given the strong evidence base for psychotherapeutic interventions for BN, it is usually best to start with one of the evidence-based psychosocial treatments. Nonetheless, medications may be considered when the patient is not responding adequately to therapy or has a comorbid psychiatric condition.

Antidepressants have been found to reduce binge eating and purging in BN. Early trials were done with tricyclics and monoamine oxidase inhibitors and generally found these medications to be effective, although side effects limited their tolerability and acceptability to patients (Agras et al. 1992; Barlow et al. 1988; Hughes et al. 1986; Leitenberg et al. 1994; Mitchell et al. 1990; Walsh et al. 1984, 1988, 1991). These classes of agents should, however, be used with caution in BN because of the potential cardiac effects of the tricyclics in possibly medically fragile patients and the difficulty patients who binge may have in complying with the dietary restrictions necessary with the monoamine oxidase inhibitors.

Newer antidepressants tend to have fewer side effects, which means patients tolerate taking them better. Fluoxetine is the most extensively researched and supported psychopharmacological treatment of BN (Aigner et al. 2011). In fact, it is the only medication approved by the U.S. Food and Drug Administration for BN. Fluoxetine has demonstrated maintenance of efficacy in reduction of binge-eating and purging behaviors, with 60 mg of fluoxetine being superior to 20 mg daily (Fluoxetine Bulimia Nervosa Collaborative Study Group 1992). This effect was found to be independent of baseline mood status (Goldstein et al. 1999). Early response to fluoxetine by week 3 is a predictor of long-term response (Sysko et al. 2010). No randomized controlled trial of fluoxetine in BN has been done with children and adolescents, but one small open trial in this population found it to be well tolerated and clinically effective (Kotler et al. 2003).

In clinical practice many different antidepressants are used, with the selective serotonin reuptake inhibitors (SSRIs) usually being the first line of treatment (Cooper and Kelland 2015). The evidence for newer-generation antidepressants other than fluoxetine is not nearly as strong as that for fluoxetine. Studies of other SSRIs, including citalopram (Leombruni et al. 2006; Sundblad et al. 2005), fluvoxamine (Brambilla et al. 1995; Fichter et al. 1996; Milano et al. 2005; Schmidt et al. 2004), and sertraline (Milano et al. 2004), have shown mixed results. Among other antidepressant drug classes, reboxetine (Fassino et al. 2004) and duloxetine (Hazen and Fava 2006) were effective in an open study and a case report, respectively. Bupropion was shown to be effective in reducing binge eating and purging, but with an unacceptably high rate of seizures, causing it to be relatively contraindicated for use in BN (Horne et al. 1988).

Various other psychotropic medications have been studied for BN. Lithium was found to not be effective (Hsu et al. 1991). A single study showed ondansetron to be effective (Faris et al. 2000). Two small open trials and one small randomized controlled trial support the use of naltrexone (Jonas and Gold 1986–1987, 1988; Marrazzi et al. 1995). Two randomized controlled trials found reduction in binge eating and purging with topiramate (Hedges et al. 2003; Hoopes et al. 2003; Nickel et al. 2005), although side effects, including sedation and cognitive effects, may limit topiramate's acceptability to patients. A current study is investigating the combination medication phentermine-topiramate for BN and BED to see if it is efficacious and if side effects are tolerable (Dalai et al. 2018).

Patients with BN commonly have comorbid psychiatric conditions that may be treated with medication; there are, however, a few issues to keep in mind in these cases. One is the rapid fluid shifts that can occur in patients who are purging or abusing laxatives, which could cause high variation in the serum concentration of medication. This would especially be of concern with medications with a narrow therapeutic window, such as lithium. Another concern is the patient's preoccupation with weight and shape. With medications that can reduce appetite, such as stimulants for attention-deficit/hyperactivity disorder, patients may be tempted to overuse medication to help with weight loss, or the appetite suppression may facilitate restricting of intake. The clinician might consider creating a contract specifying that the patient must maintain a healthy weight in order to continue taking the stimulant. Patients with eating disorders are often very reluctant to take any medications that might cause weight gain, such as atypical antipsychotics, and may find more weight-neutral options such as lurasidone more acceptable. Also, medications that increase appetite may make the patient more vulnerable to binge eating.

Treatments Illustrated

Cognitive-Behavioral Therapy—Enhanced for Bulimia Nervosa (see Case 1)

Lindsey and her therapist used CBT to address her BN. In stage 1 of treatment, the BN formulation was arrived on and Lindsey was also provided with psychoeducation regarding BN and the impact of vomiting upon her physical and mental health and thereby sports performance, as well as its ineffectiveness as a weight management/loss strategy.

Sessions in stage 1 were highly structured and included setting the agenda for session, reviewing food records, shaping Lindsey's effective use of food records, the therapist's using questioning in order to illuminate problematic problems with eating, and therapist and patient regularly referring to the personalized formulation. When Lindsey presented for treatment, she was purposefully restricting her intake except when she decided to binge eat. Lindsey was fearful of establishing regular eating; she believed it would cause uncontrollable weight gain, which would negatively impact her sports performance and her appearance. The use of psychoeducation alongside repeated reference to her personalized formulation was instrumental in supporting Lindsey's willingness to try eating three meals and one or two snacks each day. Essentially the personalized formulation stated that given the very high level of import Lindsey placed on her weight, which was again due to her belief that it was directly linked to sports performance, she used dietary restriction to attempt to control her weight. Such weight-control efforts left Lindsey hungry and feeling deprived of food, and this prompted binge-eating and purging episodes and, subsequently, renewed vows to diet better next time.

Throughout stage 1, the therapist was careful to assign and collaboratively review food records during each session. An example of Lindsey's early stage 1 food records is shown in Figure 3–1. The records allowed Lindsey to track what she was eating daily and thereby created an opportunity for both Lindsey and her therapist to observe and learn about patterns in Lindsey's eating that contributed to the binge and purge cycles. Together, they discovered that she was rarely eating breakfast and frequently avoiding snacks, and that she was eating the same meal for lunch and had been doing so for the entire semester. All meals were also notably noncalorically dense. Moreover, Lindsey was avoiding sweets, fats, and carbohydrates. She was undereating in general, but especially so given her caloric requirements for sports performance. Binge and purge cycles tended to happen in the afternoon or evening, often starting in the dining hall. She would typically binge on ice cream, bread, sweets, or cereal and also drink plenty of water, reporting that the water made purging "easier." Using the food records from Figure 3–1, the therapist asked open-ended questions to highlight that a binge episode followed insufficient intake from both the same day and the day prior. For example, Lindsey believed a recent binge started because she added croutons—a "fear food" that was a waste of calories—to her salad on Wednesday. The therapist reinforced the importance of eating the next meal or snack as scheduled after a binge-and-purge episode and thus praised Lindsey for having the yogurt and banana on Wednesday night. Lindsey worked to achieve changes in her eating patterns during stage 1. For example, therapy focused on supporting Lindsey in having breakfast each morning as well as adding a mid-morning and a mid-afternoon snack to her daily intake.

Once a regular eating pattern was largely established, therapy moved to stage 2. In this stage, Lindsey reviewed the formulation they had made during stage 1 and evaluated progress to date. The therapist and Lindsey focused their discussions on the continued importance of the regular eating as a key strategy to reduce frequency of binging and purging.

Stage 3 goals were to address factors for maintaining the BN. In Lindsey's case, the primary maintaining factor was her long-standing urge to continue to diet, which was spurred by her negative body image. She was worried that without overfocusing on food and dieting, she would gain weight and her sports performance would therefore be compromised. Thus, therapy focused on how persistent overevaluation of control over eating increased Lindsey's urge to diet, reinforced calorie counting, and ultimately led to insuf-

FIGURE 3–1. Food record example

Time	Food and drink consumed	Place	V/L	Context and Comments
Day: Tuesday				**Date:** October 10
9 am	Breakfast 1 banana 1 spoon peanut butter	Walking to class		Tired; don't want to go to class
12:30 pm	Lunch Salad: greens, tomatoes, cucumbers, peppers, grilled chicken breast	Dining Hall		Hungry
3 pm	1 granola bar and 1 Gatorade	At sport practice		Had to eat before practice; felt fat in my practice uniform; blah
4:30 pm	1 apple	After practice		
6:30 pm	Dinner Salad: greens, tomatoes, cucumbers, peppers, feta cheese, half an avocado, grilled chicken breast; ¾ cup quinoa	After practice Dining Hall		Have to work on huge presentation; don't want to

FIGURE 3–1.　Food record example *(continued)*

Time	Food and drink consumed	Place	V/L	Context and Comments
Day: Wednesday				**Date:** October 11
9 am	Breakfast 1 banana 1 spoon peanut butter	Walking to class		Presentation today; ugh; not ready
10 am	French presentation			Awful; embarrassing!!
12:30 pm	Lunch Salad: spinach, tomatoes, cucumbers, mushrooms, croutons, grilled chicken breast	Dining Hall		Regular greens looked disgusting; had to do spinach
12:45 pm		Took portions from Dining Hall and then binged in my room	V	
Maybe 1:20 pm?	2 large serving bowls of Captain Crunch cereal (about 1 box)	Same	V	Feel gross and tired so napped; missed afternoon class and practice.

FIGURE 3–1. Food record example *(continued)*

Time	Food and drink consumed	Place	V/L	Context and Comments
8 pm	2 pieces sourdough toast with extra butter 1 large serving bowl of Captain Crunch cereal 2 chocolate chip cookies 1 yogurt 1 banana	From refrigerator in room		Seems weird but was kind of hungry

ficient eating, and how insufficient eating had the biggest negative impact on Lindsey's energy levels, concentration, and sports performance. With the use of behavior and weight gain tracking, Lindsey and her therapist were able to learn that even though Lindsey did gain a modest amount of weight in therapy, this actually served to increase her energy and ultimately enhance her sport performance, which she was very pleased with. Finally, therapy progressed to stage 4, which focused on maintaining the gains she had made so far as well as minimizing the risk of relapse. Here, Lindsey and her therapist agreed that risk of relapse was greatest during Lindsey's annual competitive sport season when, historically, She had undereaten and therefore underfueled her sports performance, which prompted the binge/purge cycle. Thus, moving forward, they agreed that Lindsey would use food records throughout each future competitive season as a relapse prevention strategy. Using these records would help her stay attuned to the import of eating sufficiently. In addition, given that Lindsey was keeping the food records used in this course of therapy, she would be able to compare food intake from successful periods in therapy with the amount she was consuming during competitive season. Additional areas for future focus for Lindsey included sustaining regular eating (including incorporation of previously forbidden foods) and eating around friends and teammates during meal times rather than alone in her dorm room.

Interpersonal Psychotherapy for Bulimia Nervosa (see Case 2)

The initial phase of IPT includes assignment of the sick role, conducting the Interpersonal Inventory, identifying the interpersonal formulation, and setting the contract around therapy. The goal of IPT is to take a thorough account of current and past links between the patient's interpersonal functioning and his bulimic symptomatology. The therapist and Dillon, through the process of conducting the Interpersonal Inventory, identified that the social domain of role transitions was central to his interpersonal challenges. The category of role transitions was selected primarily because Dillon's bulimic symptoms had escalated after two recent transitions. First, he had left his home state of Michigan and moved to California 2 years earlier in order to take his current job, and second, his romantic relationship had ended 2 months prior to seeking treatment. Both of these transitions were correlated with an increase in the frequency and severity of his symptoms. Moreover, the onset of the BN symptoms in high school was subsequent to the divorce of his parents, which required him to take up a more adult role in his family after his father's departure. Since his move to the new state and job, Dillon reported that he felt isolated both at work and outside of work. He used to go out for dinner, drinks, sporting events, and concerts with friends back in Michigan. However, he felt that he was unable find and establish meaningful relationships with the individuals he met locally. Consequently, he frequently returned to his home state for visits with his mother and friends and did not spend many weekends nearby. He started rock climbing while in California but reported that he had not built friendships through the gym as of yet. He met his recent girlfriend through an online dating application, and they had dated for the past 6 months. She recently asked to end the relationship, noting that she did not feel sufficiently connected to him to continue the relationship and stating she was also interested in dating other people. In addition to loneliness, Dillon reported sadness and disappointment about his lack of connection to California in general. Despite this, Dillon really enjoyed the nature of his work and wanted to stay with his current company. The interpersonal formulation and collaboratively agreed upon treatment contract focused on role transitions, with two specific transitions in mind: 1) the end of the romantic relationship and 2) the move to California. This interpersonal formulation and contract helped set the stage for work to be done in the intermediate phase.

The goals of the intermediate phase of treatment were both to help Dillon understand the link between the social domain of role transitions and the development of BN symptomatology and to employ specific IPT techniques relevant to the social domain. Such IPT role transition–specific techniques and how they were utilized this in case are as follows:

Mourning the loss of the old role. The therapist working with Dillon encouraged him to identify and experience emotions regarding the various aspects of the old role that he may miss. In regard to the end of the romantic relationship, Dillon mourned the friendship and intimacy he would no longer experience with his previous girlfriend; the social circle she had invited him into and where he sensed he was no longer as relatively welcomed; and, importantly, the loss of someone to talk to frequently about everyday occurrences. In regard to the move to California, Dillon reported he would miss easily (i.e., without too much effort) making plans and spending time with friends in familiar hangout spots (restaurants, bars, concert venues); knowing his way around town and the "good spots" to go to where he would see familiar faces; time lost with close friends; and the potential distancing of friendships or missing out on memories they may make together while he lived out of state.

Reviewing the positive and negative aspects of both the new and old role. The therapist and Dillon worked to openly and collaboratively review both the positive and the negative aspects of each role. By doing this activity, Dillon was able to gain insight into the fact that there were aspects of his romantic relationship that he was not satisfied with and was also able to remember many things about living in Michigan that he did not like and that had initially prompted his job search in California.

Increasing patient's self-esteem toward gaining mastery in new role via discussion about feelings related to and any skills needed in order to fulfill new role. To move toward the new role of being single and adapting to life in California, Dillon collaborated with his therapist to generate a list of things for him to do that would help him gain experience in the new role and thereby increase his confidence and familiarity with it. Dillon agreed to continue to rock climb and work on building friendships at the gym, something that he had previously not tended to do. In addition, he stated he would attend the team-building events that his company hosted (e.g., dinners, outdoor activities) in order to get to know others in the office as well. Last, he stated that when he was feeling ready, he would reregister for his online dating application.

Throughout their work, Dillon's therapist was careful to highlight and inquire about the link between the BN symptoms and Dillon's interpersonal functioning. For example, at the outset of therapy, the link between Dillon's daily loneliness surrounding the relationship breakup was correlated with the onset of a binge-and-purge episode (e.g., he tended to starting binge eating right before going home from the office; evenings were a time he used to spend with his girlfriend that would now be spent alone). Throughout the course of treatment, Dillon's engagement in tasks and self-efficacy surrounding the new role (getting back into a dating application; making new friends) were associated with the reduction of binging and purging. The therapist would use questions such as "Have you noticed any connections between the decrease in binge eating and purging and how the weekend with your new work friends went?"

The termination phase of IPT focuses on readying and processing the formal end of therapy; reviewing what was accomplished during the patient's progression through treatment; identifying work to be continued after the end of treatment; and being attentive to signals of potential relapse and planning accordingly to prevent full relapse. Dillon and his therapist reviewed how his BN symptoms were linked to the two role transitions he experienced and how his symptoms improved as he worked to resolve the transition concerns, and also talked about potential early warning signals that may arise in case of another transition (relationship breakup; job transition; move to a new city; with a return to some sporadic binge-eating and purging episodes). Future work for Dillon, as collaboratively outlined by both Dillon and his therapist, included investing time and energy toward building and establishing new relationships (friendships and romantic relationships) in his new hometown.

Family-Based Therapy for Adolescent Bulimia Nervosa (see Case 3)

Prior to the initial therapy session, the therapist informed Georgia's parents of the importance of the entire family attending therapy sessions. Since Georgia's older brother was away at college, only her younger brother, Bruce, would join in addition to Georgia and both of her parents, Ron and Maggie.

FBT-BN session 1 has multiple goals, and the therapist keeps these in mind when assessing and starting therapy. For example, the therapist assesses the history of the illness and asks every family member to contribute their perspective on the development of BN and its effects on the family. To do this, the therapist uses circular questioning about how they each believe BN has impacted their loved one in all realms of her life (i.e., socially, physically, interpersonally, emotionally, familial). In addition, the therapist needs to help the family know what to expect in treatment, and this includes providing a brief description of the structure of FBT-BN (three phases; all family members at each session) as well as the collaborative nature of treatment in engaging the parents alongside their daughter to help cease the BN behaviors.

Georgia's parents reported being worried about their daughter's illness and were resolved and willing to help her, yet they were also apprehensive as they embarked on the task of facilitating establishment of healthful eating habits. Both parents stated that they were willing to commit to the process. In the consultative role, the therapist provided information about BN as well as about what other families have found helpful in their recovery process to help the family consider what approaches they feel might work best for them. In session 1, the therapist provided information about

gia used to love grilled cheese sandwiches but had been avoiding them since she was now refusing carbohydrates and cheese, citing them as a source of "wasted calories and fat." With coaching from the therapist, Georgia's parents were successful in getting her to eat half of the grilled cheese sandwich without purging thereafter. During the session, the therapist also reviewed the goals Georgia and her parents had outlined for themselves for the week prior. They reported some successes and some conundrums. Maggie had rearranged her work schedule but was having trouble figuring out how much Georgia should be eating after school. This was complicated by the fact that Georgia was still often skipping lunch at school. The therapist provided some information about how other families have approached this conundrum of not being able to supervise lunch while their adolescent is at school, including taking their son or daughter out of school temporarily to ensure foods are eaten without purging or having one parent drive to school to eat with their child (e.g., in the car). Ron stated he could drive to school and eat lunch with Maggie most days. Georgia was frustrated by the idea of eating lunch with her dad in his car but was eventually open to her parents' rationale that eating lunch would lessen her hunger at snack, which may help her eat a more appropriate snack size, thereby reducing the risk of binging and purging. The family wanted to try it out. Bruce stated he and Maggie played video and board games together after a few dinners during the week; he noted he was willing to continue to help in his role of being supportive.

During session 3, Georgia shared that she was still secretively using laxatives. Maggie and Ron asked her to give them the laxatives when they got home from session, and Georgia agreed. The therapy session then focused on how to help stop Georgia from purchasing more laxatives; Georgia said she would try, and Ron said he could monitor her spending when or if she purchased laxatives with the credit card they had given her for emergencies. The therapist also noted that Georgia's pediatrician would take labs that might implicate vomiting or laxative use if the electrolyte balance was off. The remainder of phase I continued in a similar fashion; each session was focused on helping the family collaboratively eliminate the disordered eating behaviors and empowering the parents to take the lead.

The family and therapist collaboratively decided to move onto phase II when Georgia was eating more regularly throughout the day on a consistent basis and the binge, vomiting, and laxative abuse behaviors had ceased for several weeks. During phase II of FBT-BN, Georgia and her family worked to reduce the body-checking behaviors (e.g., analyzing her body in the mirror; pinching her flesh) in order for Georgia to improve her body image. Georgia really wanted her dad to stop coming to school for lunch and reported feeling ready to commit to eating lunch everyday independently. Thus, the family transferred the responsibility to eating lunch back to Georgia. Georgia had success with this behavior over the following weeks, and thus she and her parents decided to let her independently manage her breakfasts as well. Throughout this time of transfer of responsibility back to Georgia, her weight remained stable, as did her abstinence from binging, vomiting, and laxative use. The family as a whole reported observing improvements in many areas of Georgia's life that had previously been negatively affected by the BN.

Finally, the family moved on to phase III and worked on general adolescent issues such as returning to sleepovers at friends' houses, managing the upcoming class camping trip out of town, as well as non-BN related issues such as curfew and driving privileges. Termination was a very easy process, as the family felt that they had learned how to help Georgia and that they were working effectively as a family and there was no further need for a therapist to guide them.

Common Outcomes and Complications

- Even after remission, some individuals with BN are unsure how to use the time they had been using for binge eating and purging for more productive activities, so this may be an additional therapeutic target.

- During treatment, individuals with BN need to learn to experience and tolerate fullness and not respond by purging. If fear and intolerance of fullness persistent without therapeutic intervention, then the utility of purging retains its allure.

- As time between episodes of self-induced vomiting increases, the individual may report a correlation with decreased temptation to vomit.

- Individuals with BN typically report feared foods associated with a binge onset. As patients reintegrate these foods into their lives, the clinician is encouraged to consider if they are kept within the home and how they can be reintegrated appropriately.

- Persistent negative body image is often reported by individuals with BN even after cessation of binge eating and purging. This is a likely risk factor for relapse.

- Working with athletes (e.g., professional, college, elite) with BN poses unique challenges. It is imperative that the clinician partner with a sports medicine physician in order to facilitate coordination of care.

- Impulsive behaviors (e.g., binge drinking, sexual risk taking) may emerge as recovery from binge eating and purging decreases.

- Urges to eat and a penchant to think about food frequently often persist after recovery.

- Improvement in depressive symptomatology often occurs alongside decreases in binge eating and purging even without antidepressant use or specific therapy for depression.

- BN is a maladaptive coping function, and therefore some ambivalence about giving up the behaviors is common.

Resources and Further Reading

Training Resources

CBT: Oxford Cognitive Therapy Centre: https://www.octc.co.uk/training

FBT: Training Institute for Child and Adolescent Eating Disorders: train2treat4ed.com

Fairburn CG: Cognitive Behavioral Therapy and Eating Disorders. New York, Guilford, 2008

LeGrange D, Lock J: Treating Bulimia in Adolescents: A Family Based Approach. New York, Guilford, 2007

Murphy R, Straebler S, Cooper Z, et al: Interpersonal psychotherapy (IPT) for the treatment of eating disorders, in Evidence Based Treatments for Eating Disorders. Edited by Dancyger IF, Fornari V. New York, Nova, 2009, pp 257–275

Safer DL, Telch CF, Chen E: Dialectical Behavior Therapy for Binge Eating and Bulimia. New York, Guilford, 2009

Further Reading

Agras WS, Robinson AH (eds): The Oxford Handbook of Eating Disorders, 2nd Edition. New York, Oxford University Press, 2018

Burke NL, Karam A, Tanofsky-Kraff M, et al: Interpersonal psychotherapy for the treatment of eating disorders, in The Oxford Handbook of Eating Disorders, 2nd Edition. New York, Oxford University Press, 2018, pp 287–318

Chen EY, Yiu A, Safer DL: Dialectical behavior therapy and emotion-focused therapies for eating disorders, in The Oxford Handbook of Eating Disorders, 2nd Edition. New York, Oxford University Press, 2018, pp 334–350

Fairburn CG: Overcoming Binge Eating, 2nd Edition. New York, Guilford, 2013

Grilo CM, Mitchell JE (eds): The Treatment of Eating Disorders: A Clinical Handbook. New York, Guilford, 2009

LeGrange D, Rienecke R: Family therapy for eating disorders, in The Oxford Handbook of Eating Disorders, 2nd Edition. New York, Oxford University Press, 2018, pp 319–333

Lock J, LeGrange D: Help Your Teenager Beat an Eating Disorder, 2nd Edition. New York, Guilford, 2005

Wilson GT: Cognitive-behavioral therapy for eating disorders, in The Oxford Handbook of Eating Disorders, 2nd Edition. Edited by Agras WS, Robinson AH. New York, Oxford University Press, 2018, pp 271–286

References

Academy for Eating Disorders: Eating Disorders: Critical Points for Early Recognition and Medical Risk Management in the Care of Individuals With Eating Disorders, 3rd Edition. Reston, VA, Academy for Eating Disorders, 2016

Aigner M, Treasure J, Kaye W, et al: World Federation of Societies of Biological Psychiatry (WFSBP) guidelines for the pharmacological treatment of eating disorders. World J Biol Psychiatry 12(6):400–443, 2011 21961502

American Psychiatric Association: Diagnostic and Statistical Manual of Mental Disorders, 4th Edition. Washington, DC, American Psychiatric Association, 1994

American Psychiatric Association: Diagnostic and Statistical Manual of Mental Disorders, 5th Edition. Arlington, VA, American Psychiatric Association, 2013

Agras WS, Rossiter EM, Arnow B, et al: Pharmacologic and cognitive-behavioral treatment for bulimia nervosa: a controlled comparison. Am J Psychiatry 149(1):82–87, 1992 1728190

Agras WS, Walsh T, Fairburn CG, et al: A multicenter comparison of cognitive-behavioral therapy and interpersonal psychotherapy for bulimia nervosa. Arch Gen Psychiatry 57(5):459–466, 2000 10807486

Barlow J, Blouin J, Blouin A, et al: Treatment of bulimia with desipramine: a double-blind crossover study. Can J Psychiatry 33(2):129–133, 1988 3284630

Brambilla F, Draisci A, Peirone A, et al: Combined cognitive-behavioral, psychopharmacological and nutritional therapy in bulimia nervosa. Neuropsychobiology 32(2):68–71, 1995 7477802

Bulik CM, Klump KL, Thornton L, et al: Alcohol use disorder comorbidity in eating disorders: a multicenter study. J Clin Psychiatry 65(7):1000–1006, 2004 15291691

Chui W, Safer DL, Bryson SW, et al: A comparison of ethnic groups in the treatment of bulimia nervosa. Eat Behav 8(4):485–491, 2007 17950937

Cooper M, Kelland H: Medication and psychotherapy in eating disorders: is there a gap between research and practice? J Eat Disord 3:45, 2015 26629344

Dalai SS, Adler S, Najarian T, et al: Study protocol and rationale for a randomized double-blinded crossover trial of phentermine-topiramate ER versus placebo to treat binge eating disorder and bulimia nervosa. Contemp Clin Trials 64:173–178, 2018 29038069

Fairburn CG: Overcoming Binge Eating. New York, Guilford, 1995

Fairburn CG: Overcoming Binge Eating, 2nd Edition. New York, Guilford, 2013

Fairburn CG, Cooper Z: The Eating Disorder Examination, 12th edition, in Binge Eating: Nature, Assessment, and Treatment. Edited by Fairburn CG, Wilson GT. New York, Guilford, 1993, pp 317–360

Fairburn CG, Cooper Z, Shafran R: Enhanced cognitive behavioral therapy for eating disorders ("CBT-E"): an overview, in Cognitive Behavioral Therapy and Eating Disorders. Edited by Fairburn CG. New York, Guilford, 2008, pp 23–34

Fairburn CG, Cooper Z, Doll HA, et al: Transdiagnostic cognitive-behavioral therapy for patients with eating disorders: a two-site trial with 60-week follow-up. Am J Psychiatry 166(3):311–319, 2009 19074978

Fairburn CG, Bailey-Straebler S, Basden S, et al: A transdiagnostic comparison of enhanced cognitive behaviour therapy (CBT-E) and interpersonal psychotherapy in the treatment of eating disorders. Behav Res Ther 70:64–71, 2015 26000757

Faris PL, Kim SW, Meller WH, et al: Effect of decreasing afferent vagal activity with ondansetron on symptoms of bulimia nervosa: a randomised, double-blind trial. Lancet 355(9206):792–797, 2000 10711927

Fassino S, Daga GA, Boggio S, et al: Use of reboxetine in bulimia nervosa: a pilot study. J Psychopharmacol 18(3):423–428, 2004 15358988

Fichter MM, Krüger R, Rief W, et al: Fluvoxamine in prevention of relapse in bulimia nervosa: effects on eating-specific psychopathology. J Clin Psychopharmacol 16(1):9–18, 1996 8834413

Fluoxetine Bulimia Nervosa Collaborative Study Group: Fluoxetine in the treatment of bulimia nervosa. A multicenter, placebo-controlled, double-blind trial. Arch Gen Psychiatry 49(2):139–147, 1992 1550466

Goldbloom DS, Olmsted M, Davis R, et al: A randomized controlled trial of fluoxetine and cognitive behavioral therapy for bulimia nervosa: short-term outcome. Behav Res Ther 35(9):803–811, 1997 9299800

Golden NH, Katzman DK, Sawyer SM, et al: Update on the medical management of eating disorders in adolescents. J Adolesc Health 56(4):370–375, 2015 25659201

Goldstein DJ, Wilson MG, Ascroft RC, et al: Effectiveness of fluoxetine therapy in bulimia nervosa regardless of comorbid depression. Int J Eat Disord 25(1):19–27, 1999 9924649

Guerrieri R, Nederkoorn C, Jansen A: How impulsiveness and variety influence food intake in a sample of healthy women. Appetite 48(1):119–122, 2007 16959373

Hazen E, Fava M: Successful treatment with duloxetine in a case of treatment refractory bulimia nervosa: a case report. J Psychopharmacol 20(5):723–724, 2006 16401659

Hedges DW, Reimherr FW, Hoopes SP, et al: Treatment of bulimia nervosa with topiramate in a randomized, double-blind, placebo-controlled trial, part 2: improvement in psychiatric measures. J Clin Psychiatry 64(12):1449–1454, 2003 14728106

Hoopes SP, Reimherr FW, Hedges DW, et al: Treatment of bulimia nervosa with topiramate in a randomized, double-blind, placebo-controlled trial, part 1: improvement in binge and purge measures. J Clin Psychiatry 64(11):1335–1341, 2003 14658948

Horne RL, Ferguson JM, Pope HG Jr, et al: Treatment of bulimia with bupropion: a multicenter controlled trial. J Clin Psychiatry 49(7):262–266, 1988 3134343

Hsu LKG, Clement L, Santhouse R, et al: Treatment of bulimia nervosa with lithium carbonate. A controlled study. J Nerv Ment Dis 179(6):351–355, 1991 1904908

Hudson J, Hiripi E, Pop E, et al: The prevalence and correlates of eating disorder in the national comorbidity survey replication. Biol Psychiatry 61(3):1–32, 2008 16815322

Hughes PL, Wells LA, Cunningham CJ, et al: Treating bulimia with desipramine. A double-blind, placebo-controlled study. Arch Gen Psychiatry 43(2):182–186, 1986 3511878

Jonas JM, Gold MS: Treatment of antidepressant-resistant bulimia with naltrexone. Int J Psychiatry Med 16(4):305–309, 1986–1987 3557806

Jonas JM, Gold MS: The use of opiate antagonists in treating bulimia: a study of low-dose versus high-dose naltrexone. Psychiatry Res 24(2):195–199, 1988 2841709

Karhunen LJ, Lappalainen RI, Tammela L, et al: Subjective and physiological cephalic phase responses to food in obese binge-eating women. Int J Eat Disord 21(4):321–328, 1997 9138042

Kotler LA, Devlin MJ, Davies M, et al: An open trial of fluoxetine for adolescents with bulimia nervosa. J Child Adolesc Psychopharmacol 13(3):329–335, 2003 14642021

Leitenberg H, Rosen JC, Wolf J, et al: Comparison of cognitive-behavior therapy and desipramine in the treatment of bulimia nervosa. Behav Res Ther 32(1):37–45, 1994 8135721

Le Grange D, Lock J: Treating Bulimia in Adolescents: A Family Based Approach. New York, Guilford, 2007

Le Grange D, Lock J, Agras WS, et al: Randomized clinical trial of family based treatment and cognitive-behavioral therapy for adolescent bulimia nervosa. J Am Acad Child Adolesc Psychiatry 54(11):886–894, 2015 26506579

Leombruni P, Amianto F, Delsedime N, et al: Citalopram versus fluoxetine for the treatment of patients with bulimia nervosa: a single-blind randomized controlled trial. Adv Ther 23(3):481–494, 2006 16912031

Linehan MM: Cognitive Behavioral Therapy of Borderline Personality Disorder. New York, Guilford, 1993a

Linehan MM: Skills Training Manual for Treating Borderline Personality Disorder. New York, Guilford, 1993b

Loxton NJ, Dawe S: How do dysfunctional eating and hazardous drinking women perform on behavioural measures of reward and punishment sensitivity? Pers Individ Dif 42(6):1163–1172, 2007

Markowitz JC, Skodol AE, Bleiberg K: Interpersonal psychotherapy for borderline personality disorder: possible mechanisms of change. J Clin Psychol 62(4):431–444, 2006 16470711

Marrazzi MA, Bacon JP, Kinzie J, et al: Naltrexone use in the treatment of anorexia nervosa and bulimia nervosa. Int Clin Psychopharmacol 10(3):163–172, 1995 8675969

Milano W, Petrella C, Sabatino C, et al: Treatment of bulimia nervosa with sertraline: a randomized controlled trial. Adv Ther 21(4):232–237, 2004 15605617

Milano W, Siano C, Putrella C, et al: Treatment of bulimia nervosa with fluvoxamine: a randomized controlled trial. Adv Ther 22(3):278–283, 2005 16236688

Mitchell JE, Pyle RL, Eckert ED, et al: A comparison study of antidepressants and structured intensive group psychotherapy in the treatment of bulimia nervosa. Arch Gen Psychiatry 47(2):149–157, 1990 2405806

National Institute for Health and Care Excellence: Eating Disorders: Recognition and Treatment. London, British Psychological Society, 2017

Nickel C, Tritt K, Muehlbacher M, et al: Topiramate treatment in bulimia nervosa patients: a randomized, double-blind, placebo-controlled trial. Int J Eat Disord 38(4):295–300, 2005 16231337

Penas-Lledó E, Waller G: Bulimic psychopathology and impulsive behaviors among nonclinical women. Int J Eat Disord 29(1):71–75, 2001 11135336

Perkins SJ, Murphy R, Schmidt U, et al: Self-help and guided self-help for eating disorders. Cochrane Database Syst Rev (3):CD004191, 2006 16856036

Pidcock BW, Fischer JL, Forthun LF, et al: Hispanic and Anglo college women's risk factors for substance use and eating disorders. Addict Behav 25(5):705–723, 2000 11023013

Polivy J, Herman CP: Etiology of binge eating: psychological mechanisms, in Binge Eating: Nature, Assessment, and Treatment. Edited by Fairburn CG, Wilson GT. New York, Guilford, 1993, pp 173–205

Poulsen S, Lunn S, Daniel SIF, et al: A randomized controlled trial of psychoanalytic psychotherapy or cognitive-behavioral therapy for bulimia nervosa. Am J Psychiatry 171(1):109–116, 2014 24275909

Safer DL, Telch CF, Agras WS: Dialectical behavior therapy for bulimia nervosa. Am J Psychiatry 158(4):632–634, 2001 11282700

Schmidt U, Cooper PJ, Essers H, et al: Fluvoxamine and graded psychotherapy in the treatment of bulimia nervosa: a randomized, double-blind, placebo-controlled, multicenter study of short-term and long-term pharmacotherapy combined with a stepped care approach to psychotherapy. J Clin Psychopharmacol 24(5):549–552, 2004 15349014

Schmidt U, Lee S, Beecham J, et al: A randomized controlled trial of family therapy and cognitive behavior therapy guided self-care for adolescents with bulimia nervosa and related disorders. Am J Psychiatry 164(4):591–598, 2007 17403972

Stefano SC, Bacaltchuk J, Blay SL, et al: Self-help treatments for disorders of recurrent binge eating: a systematic review. Acta Psychiatr Scand 113(6):452–459, 2006 16677221

Sundblad C, Landén M, Eriksson T, et al: Effects of the androgen antagonist flutamide and the serotonin reuptake inhibitor citalopram in bulimia nervosa: a placebo-controlled pilot study. J Clin Psychopharmacol 25(1):85–88, 2005 15643104

Swanson SA, Crow SJ, Le Grange D, et al: Prevalence and correlates of eating disorders in adolescents. Results from the national comorbidity survey replication adolescent supplement. Arch Gen Psychiatry 68(7):714–723, 2011 21383252

Sysko R, Sha N, Wang Y, et al: Early response to antidepressant treatment in bulimia nervosa. Psychol Med 40(6):999–1005, 2010 20441691

Tanofsky-Kraff M, Wilfley DE: Interpersonal psychotherapy (IPT) for bulimia nervosa and binge eating disorder, in The Treatment of Eating Disorders. Edited by Grilo C, Mitchell J. New York, Guilford, 2009, pp 271–293

Vervaet M, Audenaert K, van Heeringen C: Cognitive and behavioural characteristics are associated with personality dimensions in patients with eating disorders. Eur Eat Disord Rev 11(5):363–378, 2003

Walsh BT, Stewart JW, Roose SP, et al: Treatment of bulimia with phenelzine. A double-blind, placebo-controlled study. Arch Gen Psychiatry 41(11):1105–1109, 1984 6388524

Walsh BT, Gladis M, Roose SP, et al: Phenelzine vs placebo in 50 patients with bulimia. Arch Gen Psychiatry 45(5):471–475, 1988 3282482

Walsh BT, Hadigan CM, Devlin MJ, et al: Long-term outcome of antidepressant treatment for bulimia nervosa. Am J Psychiatry 148(9):1206–1212, 1991 1882999

Walsh BT, Wilson GT, Loeb KL, et al: Medication and psychotherapy in the treatment of bulimia nervosa. Am J Psychiatry 154(4):523–531, 1997 9090340

Wilfley DE, Wilson GT, Agras WS: A multisite randomized controlled trial of interpersonal psychotherapy, behavioral weight loss, and guided self-help in the treatment of overweight individuals with binge eating disorder. Paper presented at the fourteenth annual meeting of the Eating Disorders Research Society, Montreal, Canada, October 2008

Wilson GT, Grilo CM, Vitousek KM: Psychological treatment of eating disorders. Am Psychol 62(3):199–216, 2007 17469898

Wilson GT: Cognitive behavioral therapy for eating disorders, in Handbook for Eating Disorders. Edited by Agras WS. New York, Oxford University Press, 2010, pp 331–347

Chapter 4

Binge-Eating Disorder

Cristin D. Runfola, Ph.D.
Sarah Adler, Psy.D.
Debra L. Safer, M.D.

Introduction

Binge-eating disorder (BED) was first formally described in 1959 by Albert Stunkard, who identified it as a pattern of abnormal eating found in patients with obesity. BED was not included in the *Diagnostic and Statistical Manual of Mental Disorders,* however, until the fourth edition (DSM-IV; American Psychiatric Association 1994). At that point it was introduced as a provisional diagnosis requiring further study within the category "Eating Disorder Not Otherwise Specified" (EDNOS). BED was officially added as a distinct standalone diagnosis in the fifth edition (DSM-5; American Psychiatric Association 2013).

Data accumulated between DSM-IV and DSM-5 led to the establishment of less stringent criteria for binge frequency and symptom duration in the later version. Currently, a diagnosis of BED requires the presence of recurrent (once weekly or more often) binge-eating episodes characterized by the consumption of objectively large amounts of food (e.g., beyond what is typical given the context) over a discrete period of time (e.g., 2 hours) *and* a sense of loss of control over eating during the episode. *Loss of control* means not being able to stop eating or control what or how much one has eaten. Episodes must also be associated with *three or more* features: eating rapidly, eating until the point of being uncomfortably full, eating despite lack of physical hunger, eating alone due to embarrassment about what or how much one is eating, or feeling disgust, depression, or guilt after eating. Marked distress associated with the binge-eating behavior must be reported, in addition to the behavior lasting 3 months or more.

BED severity specifiers are included in DSM-5 based on the frequency, per week, of binge-eating episodes (e.g., mild [1–3], moderate [4–7], severe [5–13], and extreme [≥14]) and can be increased based on functional disability or related symptomatology as clinically indicated (American Psychiatric Association 2013). For example, although not a diagnostic criterion of BED, overvaluation of shape and weight on self-worth has been associated with greater severity of eating pathology and psychological distress (Grilo 2013). Similarly, the presence of emotional eating in obese individuals with BED correlates with the severity of binge eating and general eating psychopathology (Masheb and Grilo 2006; Ricca et al. 2009). The existence of such correlates suggests a worse clinical profile and subsequent increase in the severity specifier. However, there is currently a lack of consensus regarding the validity of the BED specifier (Dakanalis et al. 2017; Gianini et al. 2017; Nakai et al. 2017; Smith et al. 2017b).

Key Diagnostic Checklist

❏ Binge eating (large amount of food plus loss of control) occurring at least once per week for a minimum of 3 months in the absence of compensatory behaviors (American Psychiatric Association 2015). In children and adolescents, loss of control over eating appears a better clinical marker of binge eating than the amount of food consumed (Marcus and Kalarchian 2003).

❏ Association of binge eating with at least three of five other features, including eating much more quickly than normal, eating until the point of physical discomfort, eating despite lack of physical hunger, eating alone due to embarrassment about one's amount of food intake, and feeling disgust, depression, or guilt after binge eating.

❏ Distress due to binge-eating symptoms.

❏ Severity of mild to extreme according to frequency of binge-eating episodes per week. It has been recommended to use a lower threshold when making the diagnosis in children and adolescents, specifically to once per month over a 3-month period (Bravender et al. 2007), based on evidence of developmental differences in reports of binge eating between youth and adults (Peebles et al. 2006).

Diagnostic Rule Outs

- *Other eating disorders.* The recurrent presence of inappropriate compensatory behaviors, such as purging, excessive exercise, or laxative abuse, is uncharacteristic of binge-eating disorder (American Psychiatric Association 2013). If these behaviors are present, another eating disorder diagnosis besides BED should be considered, namely, bulimia nervosa; anorexia nervosa, binge eating/purging type; or other specified feeding and eating disorder (OSFED; e.g., purging disorder).

- *Mood disorders.* Although increased appetite and unintentional weight gain are associated with major depressive disorder and bipolar disorder, the increased eating in this context must be accompanied by a loss of control over eating—a characteristic of binge eating—to receive a BED diagnosis (American Psychiatric Association 2013; Wilfley et al. 2016). The co-occurrence of BED and mood disorder is high.

- *Borderline personality disorder.* Binge eating is listed as an example of an impulsive behavior under the diagnostic criteria for borderline personality disorder. If full criteria are met for both BED and borderline personality, both diagnoses should be given.

- *Obesity.* Not everyone who has obesity has binge-eating behavior, and vice versa. Obesity is not a diagnostic criterion of BED. If eating disorder symptoms are not present in the individual with obesity, only a diagnosis of obesity is appropriate.

Epidemiology and Risk Factors

Epidemiology

- Onset of BED is typically around early adulthood, with a mean age at onset of 23.3 years (Kessler et al. 2013).
- BED is the most common of the eating disorders. Among adults in the United States, lifetime prevalence estimates range from 1.52% to 2.6% and 12-month prevalence estimates range from 1.2% to 1.64% depending on study and

diagnostic criteria (DSM-IV vs. DSM-5). In adolescents, the lifetime prevalence is 2.3% in females and 0.8% in males (Swanson et al. 2011).

- The prevalence of BED is higher among certain groups of adult individuals, such as individuals with obesity (36.2%–42.4%; Wilfley et al. 2016), individuals seeking treatment for weight control (13%–27%; Wilfley et al. 2016), and persons undergoing bariatric surgery (~49%; de Zwaan et al. 2003; Niego et al. 2007).

- BED may be slightly more common among ethnic minority groups than among non-Latino whites (Kornstein 2017) and slightly more common in women than in men. The gender ratio (female:male) is about 3:2 in adults (Hudson et al. 2007). Biological and sociocultural factors may influence this gender discrepancy. For example, variations in estrogen levels have been observed to impact genetic risks for eating disorders in girls at puberty (Klump 2013), suggesting ovarian hormones may play a role in BED risk at key periods of hormone change (Baker and Runfola 2016). Among sociocultural factors, increased exposure to dieting, peer pressure, and overvaluation of the "thin ideal" among females are believed to preferentially increase risk for eating disorders among women (Slevec and Tiggemann 2011; Urquhart and Mihalynuk 2011).

Risk Factors

- BED is heritable and clusters in families (Hudson et al. 2006; Javaras et al. 2008; Mitchell et al. 2010). Correlational and prospective studies suggest various other specific risk factors may exist—for example, parental perception of childhood overweight, familial eating problems, preadolescent loss of control eating, body dissatisfaction, negative affect associated with clinical depression, and adverse life experiences (Ambrogne 2017; Blostein et al. 2017; Palmisano et al. 2016; Tanofsky-Kraff et al. 2011). Generally, the etiology of BED is multifactorial and precipitated by the interaction of several risk factors, including genetic, biological, psychological, environmental, cultural, and sociological variables. See Culbert et al. 2015 for a comprehensive review.

Common Comorbidities

Medical

- *Obesity.* BED is associated with the development of obesity, increased medical morbidity, and increased mortality (Fichter and Quadflieg 2016; Kessler et al. 2013). About 42.4% of individuals with BED have obesity (i.e., body mass index > 30 kg/m^2; Hudson et al. 2007). Furthermore, BED independently increases risk for the development of certain components of the metabolic syndrome, type 2 diabetes, hypertension, and dyslipidemia, above and beyond those accounted for by obesity alone (Hudson et al. 2010).

- *Other medical problems.* Other medical problems associated with BED include pain conditions, sleep disorders, fibromyalgia, somatic illness, and gastrointestinal symptoms (Citrome 2017; Olguin et al. 2017; Thornton et al. 2017). Among women with BED or binge-eating behavior, associations have been observed with pregnancy complications, menstrual dysfunction, and polycystic ovary syndrome (Olguin et al. 2017). Preliminary data suggest that the cardiovascular system, reproductive system, and cortisol response might be affected by BED (Mitchell 2016; Thornton et al. 2017).

Psychiatric

- *General.* BED commonly co-occurs with other psychiatric disorders, irrespective of weight status (Guerdjikova et al. 2017a). In a clinical sample, up to about 74% of adult patients with BED were found to have at least one psychiatric disorder in their lifetime and about 43% to have a current psychiatric disorder (Grilo et al. 2009). Rates of major depressive disorder, posttraumatic stress disorder, generalized anxiety disorder, obsessive-compulsive disorder, panic attacks, impulse-control disorders, and substance abuse are all higher in individuals with BED.

- *Personality disorders.* Personality disorders are also more common in adults with BED than in those without the disorder, with both Cluster B (e.g., borderline personality disorder) and Cluster C (e.g., avoidant personality disorder, obsessive-compulsive personality disorder) disorders significantly more prevalent (Specker et al. 1994). The degree of co-occurring psychological disorders is related to binge eating severity rather than degree of overweight (Citrome 2017).

- *Intra- and interpersonal stresses.* Significant intra- and interpersonal stresses are associated with BED (Arcelus et al. 2013). Women with BED tend more to view interpersonal relationships as stressful (Riener et al. 2006), which may be due to interpersonal sensitivity, paranoid ideas (Fandiño et al. 2010), difficulties with boundary setting, and overinvolvement in social relationships (Ansell et al. 2012).

- *Impaired quality of life and functional disability.* BED is also associated with impaired quality of life and functional disability (Pawaskar et al. 2017; Wilfley et al. 2016). For example, in a population-based sample, up to 63% of individuals with BED reported functional impairment in domains of either work, home, social life, or personal life in the previous year, with 18.5% noting severe impairment (Hudson et al. 2007).

- *Suicidal ideation and behavior.* Suicidal behavior is elevated in individuals with BED relative to the general population (Smith et al. 2017a). About 21%–23% of adults with BED or OSFED report current suicidal ideation (Favaro and Santonastaso 1997; Milos et al. 2004). Preliminary data on temporal patterns show most adolescents experience suicidality onset following BED onset, whereas most adults experienced suicidality onset prior to BED onset (Forrest et al. 2017).

Clinical Presentations

Case 1: Valerie

Valerie is a 21-year-old female with a body mass index (BMI) of 23 kg/m² self-referred to a university psychiatry clinic at the suggestion of her parents. She had been diagnosed with anorexia nervosa at age 13. She was successfully restored to a healthy weight after 1 year of family-based therapy. She reported minimal concerns about weight and shape since then and appeared to be in full recovery until 6 months before reinitiating treatment. As a member of her university diving team, she suffered an injury and found herself unable to train and compete. This led to a significant amount of free time, and she reported the onset of behaviors during periods when she used to be training with her teammates. Her increase in caloric intake and lack of physical activity led to weight gain, which was noticed by her parents and teammates—who would comment on the change in her body and warn her to "stay healthy" so she could continue to compete. The patient began to worry that her weight would impact her return to the team, and she became increasingly focused on her body. Additionally, she began to worry that she might not be accepted if she was "fat" or "not athletic," and to question her value outside being an athlete. These concerns regarding weight and the change in her shape led to a resurgence of caloric restriction, where she reported skipping breakfast and eating a dramatically reduced lunch portion. The patient reported that she would feel exhausted and "ravenous" by dinner, and she would be unable to control her portion sizes. For example, about **four or five times a week,** she reported **losing control and eating large quantities of food** (e.g., three bags of microwave popcorn) **rapidly, over the course of 15–20 minutes.** She would **eat alone** in her dorm room to avoid the embarrassment of being seen. Afterward she would feel **intense guilt and shame** about her behavior, telling herself that she was disgusting and that she would never be able to be on the diving team again. She endorsed **terrible distress associated with her behavior.**

Case 2: Samantha

Samantha is a 45-year-old married female with a BMI of about 31 kg/m^2 presenting to your office for help with her "out-of-control eating," depressed mood, and weight. She began to experience loss-of-control episodes in her early teens that were triggered by interpersonal difficulties with her peers, leaving her feeling alienated—as though she did not fit in. She reports that she learned to compare herself with others constantly, which would leave her feeling sad and "less than." She found that eating numbed some of these feelings. She also reports that for about a year she vomited after she overate but found it too time consuming and difficult to continue on a regular basis. She has also suffered from recurrent depression since high school and hypothesized that she may even have been depressed as a small child. She denies a history of substance abuse except for what might have been alcohol abuse in college, when her binge frequency reduced. The patient reports that she still engaged in some emotional overeating during this period but was able to maintain her weight with exercise. She also reports that her weight increased after the birth of her first child 13 years ago. Transitioning from working to becoming a stay-at-home mother of three, she reports having had less time to exercise or to prepare "healthy foods." Additionally, eating regularly became sporadic.

She reports that her husband travels a great deal, and she resents his lack of involvement, which creates tension in the marriage, resentment, and anger, which she would attempt to "eat away" to avoid conflict. This has led to an increase in binge episode frequency with the following pattern: In front of her family she limits herself to a "normal" meal but continues to eat in an **"out-of-control manner"** throughout clean-up and until bedtime **nearly every night.** She reports eating the equivalent of another two full meals. For example, she might have a hamburger and salad for dinner but then another two or three hamburgers with buns, three-quarters of a family sized bag of potato chips, and one-half to three-quarters of a pint of ice cream. Her after-dinner **eating is conducted secretively,** when she is alone cleaning up the kitchen or after her family has gone to bed, because she feels embarrassed to have anyone else see how much she is consuming. She describes **eating even when not physically hungry.** By the time she is in bed, she feels **intense disgust with herself and guilt.** She reports feeling **extremely distressed** by her eating behavior. Additionally, the patient reports occasional panic attacks and diffuse anxiety that are primarily focused on eating-related issues or social situations. Her low mood is primarily driven by interpersonal conflict with her husband. She denies a history consistent with obsessive-compulsive disorder or posttraumatic stress disorder.

Evidence-Based Psychosocial Outpatient Treatments for Binge-Eating Disorder

Adults

Cognitive-behavioral therapy (Fairburn et al. 2008)—Level 1 (established treatment)

Interpersonal psychotherapy (IPT) (Rieger et al. 2010)—Level 2 (probably efficacious)

Dialectical behavior therapy (DBT) (Safer et al. 2009)—Level 2 (probably efficacious)

Behavioral weight loss (BWL) (Peat et al. 2017—Level 2 (probably efficacious)

Children and Adolescents

Interpersonal psychotherapy (Rieger et al. 2010)—Level 2 (possibly efficacious)

Treatment Settings

Treatment for BED can occur at varying levels of care depending on severity of symptoms and treatment responses. From least intensive to most intensive, levels of care include guided self-help, outpatient, intensive outpatient/partial hospitalization/day treatment, inpatient treatment, or residential care. Across levels of care, treatment may include psychotherapy, pharmacotherapy, nutritional counseling, and medical monitoring.

Favorable outcomes for cognitive-behavioral therapy (CBT)–guided self-help programs for adult BED have been reported (Peat et al. 2017), especially for cases in which the BED is of mild severity and there is no comorbidity (Vocks et al. 2010). The addition of a smartphone application with CBT–guided self-help may result in improved adherence and more rapid decreases in binge eating frequency by the end of treatment (Hildebrandt et al. 2017). Guided self-help outperforms unguided (or pure) self-help (Wilson et al. 2000). In youth with BED, preliminary data suggest that internet-facilitated CBT self-help treatment may also facilitate proportional weight loss (Jones et al. 2008). However, whether these treatments can be delivered in "real-world" settings is not yet known; lack of insurance coverage for phone or video-conferencing sessions may pose a treatment barrier.

Most treatment for BED occurs in an outpatient setting. Data suggest that even complex or "challenging" patients with obesity and high rates of psychiatric comorbidity can be treated for BED effectively in an outpatient setting following a manualized protocol (Grilo 2017). On the basis of anecdotal reports, some clinicians refer patients to more intensive treatment programs following a failed course of outpatient treatment or in the context of severe comorbidity (e.g., suicidal ideation). However, there are insufficient data to support higher levels of care for BED at this time (Peat et al. 2017).

A number of applications for mobile devices exist as self-help tools or as an enhancement of existing eating disorder treatments (Fairburn and Rothwell 2015).

Treatments

Various psychological, behavioral, and pharmacological interventions have been tried to reduce BED symptomatology. In the following subsections we briefly summarize the core interventions for BED as well as therapy outcome evidence grades based on American Psychological Association guidelines (Silverman and Hinshaw 2008).

Psychological and Behavioral Interventions

Psychological and behavioral interventions with the strongest evidence base for the treatment of adult BED include CBT (Level 1), IPT (Level 2), DBT (Level 2), and BWL (Level 3); (Berkman et al. 2015; Grilo 2017; Peat et al. 2017). Each of these behavioral therapies shows solid evidence for obtaining abstinence from binge eating with differences in time of response, acceptability, long-term maintenance of symptom reduction, and the number of replication studies. Group acceptance-based behavioral therapy (ABBT) and cognitive-behavioral couple-based therapy for BED (called UNITE) also appear promising for adult BED (Level 4). The vast majority of randomized controlled trials evaluating eating disorders have assessed interventions for adult women, and many of these interventions have yet to be tested or adapted in adolescents. There are no randomized controlled trials for adolescent BED to date. As with all psychotherapies, determining which intervention to use requires a clinical conceptualization of the case presentation congruent with the treatment model.

Cognitive-Behavioral Therapy

CBT (Fairburn 1995; Marcus 1997) is based on a theoretical model that posits certain cognitions and attitudes regarding the importance of shape and weight influence how individuals feel about their bodies and their self-worth, and these attitudes can lead to maladaptive or restrictive dieting, which (in turn) can lead to binge eating. Hence, CBT focuses on normalizing eating patterns (i.e., decreasing dietary restraint, reducing binge eating); identifying and challenging negative thoughts about eating, weight, and shape to address irrational cognitions; reducing overvaluation of weight/shape on self-worth while improving body image; and teaching problem-solving skills to better manage triggering events, slips, and relapses. CBT for BED has been effectively delivered in 1-hour sessions over 12–24 weeks (Fairburn 2008) in individual or group formats (Grenon et al. 2017) and online (Wagner et al. 2016). For adults, CBT reliably produces short- and long-term reductions in binge-eating frequency and associated psychopathology, with greater than 50% abstinence rates by end of treatment through up to 48 months of follow-up (Grilo 2017). Weight does not reduce significantly over the course of treatment, but adding exercise and biweekly maintenance to CBT improves weight loss outcomes (Pendleton et al. 2002). Data from the Agency for Healthcare Quality and Research evidence-based review of the efficacy of BED treatment of all the existing interventions (Berkman et al. 2015) indicate that therapist-led CBT for BED has the strongest evidence base. Practice guidelines have described CBT in either individual or group format as a first-line treatment for BED (National Institute for Health and Care Excellence 2017; Wilson and Shafran 2005; Yager et al. 2012).

Interpersonal Psychotherapy

IPT (Wilfley et al. 1993, 2002; Tanofsky-Kraff et al. 2010) aims to resolve interpersonal problems known to maintain disordered eating. IPT consists of one 2-hour session and 18 hour-long sessions delivered weekly to biweekly over three phases focused on improving social functioning across four domains: interpersonal deficits, role conflicts, role transitions, and grief or loss. Patients learn how to manage emotions effectively, improve interpersonal experiences, and enhance psychosocial functioning. For adults, IPT reliably produces short- and long-term reductions in binge eating frequency and associated psychopathology (Grilo 2017). Studies generally find rates of binge-eating abstinence (defined as no binge-eating episodes within the past month) of approximately 50%–60% by end of treatment, with these rates well maintained through follow-up periods up to 24 months. IPT in adults with BED appears particularly effective in racial/ethnic minorities, patients with more severe symptomology, and patients with low self-esteem, as compared with CBT (Wilson et al. 2010). Although IPT has not yet been tested in adolescents with BED, preliminary pilot work suggests that IPT is feasible in adolescents with bulimia nervosa and may reduce frequency of loss of control over eating as well as prevent excess weight gain (Tanofsky-Kraff et al. 2010; Wilfley et al. 2002).

Dialectical Behavior Therapy

DBT, based on the affect-regulation model, conceptualizes binge eating as a maladaptive strategy for managing unpleasant emotional states. In individual or group format (typically 20 sessions), the DBT therapist acts as a "coach," primarily helping patients with BED develop skills to manage negative emotions (Safer et al. 2007). As with all DBT programs, the intervention helps patients build skills in multiple domains: mindfulness, distress tolerance, emotion regulation, and interpersonal effectiveness. Although DBT has a smaller evidence base than CBT and IPT, accumulating evidence suggests DBT is an efficacious treatment for adults with BED (Safer et al. 2010; Telch et al. 2000, 2001), with promising binge-eating abstinence rates found posttreatment (Grilo 2017). In one randomized controlled trial comparing group DBT for BED (DBT-BED) with an active comparison group therapy, significantly higher rates of binge-eating abstinence were observed at posttreatment (64% for DBT-BED vs. 36% active group therapy) but not at follow-up periods (e.g., 12-month follow-up abstinence rate 64% for DBT-BED vs. 56% for active group therapy), suggesting that group DBT-BED may decrease binge eating more quickly than nonspecialized group therapy. Importantly, DBT-BED showed significantly fewer dropouts than active comparison group therapy. Preliminary case studies suggest that DBT-BED can be used in a guided self-help format (Masson et al. 2013) and can also be adapted and applied to adolescent BED (Safer et al. 2007).

Behavioral Weight Loss

BWL treatment (Agras et al. 1994; Marcus et al. 1995) addresses chaotic eating patterns and the overconsumption of calories characteristic of BED patients with obesity. It is a structured behavioral lifestyle approach that focuses specifically on normalizing and structuring eating and increasing physical activity. It has been implemented with various populations, such as diabetes patients, with some clinician protocols and patient "tool kits" available online (Wing et al. 2004). BWL appears less effective than CBT at reducing binge-eating frequency (Grilo et al. 2011) and achieving long-term remission rates (Grilo 2017). However, in contrast to CBT, IPT, and DBT, which do not produce significant weight loss (McElroy et al. 2015), BWL has been shown to produce modest weight loss at least in the short term (Grilo et al. 2011). In a 2-year follow-up study comparing BWL with IPT and CBT–guided self-help, significant differences in weight loss across treatments observed posttreatment were no longer apparent (Wilson et al. 2010). Thus, use of BWL should be carefully considered given the lower rates of reduction in binge behaviors that are a significant part of the distress associated with BED. Additionally, approximately 60% of individuals with BED report an overvaluation of shape and weight, suggesting careful evaluation of the use of treatments that focus on weight loss as a main outcome.

Experimental Interventions

Other exploratory interventions exist. The use of virtual and augmented realities (VR and AR) in the treatment of eating disorders is gaining interest. Randomized controlled trials have shown that the efficacy of VR-enhanced CBT is superior to that of CBT alone in the treatment of eating disorders (Cesa et al. 2013; Manzoni et al. 2016; Marco et al. 2013). Overall, data suggest VR-enhanced evidence-based treatments may result in faster effects with better maintenance than standard treatment alone (Ferrer-García et al. 2017; Maldonado et al. 2018; Marco et al. 2013; Perpiñá et al. 2004; Riva et al. 2003, 2004). Two other exploratory interventions—10-session group ABBT (Juarascio et al. 2017) and a 22-session intervention for BED called UNITE (Runfola et al. 2016)—have been developed. On the basis of open pilot trials, these treatments appear to be promising for achieving binge abstinence as well as reducing binge-eating frequency and related symptomatology, including at follow-up. ABBT and UNITE also resulted in a significant reduction of depression symptoms and improvement in emotion regulation over the course of treatment. Because the findings are based on small sample sizes and no randomized controlled trials exist, these results should be interpreted with caution.

Finally, mindfulness-based interventions for BED are being studied (Kristeller and Hallett 1999; Ruffault et al. 2016). The primary aim of these interventions is to build nonjudgmental and moment-to-moment attention to the present experience. One program has been evaluated within a BED sample, namely, mindfulness-based eating awareness training (MB-EAT; Kristeller and Hallett 1999), consisting of 10 group sessions focused on training in mindfulness meditation and guided mindfulness practices to address the core issues of BED. The primary focus is to help participants better control responses to emotional states, make more conscious food choices, foster awareness of hunger and satiety cues, and cultivate self-acceptance. Preliminary studies show promise for reducing binge-eating episodes, improving one's sense of control related to eating, and reducing depression symptomatology.

Pharmacological Treatments

While psychological treatments are generally considered a mainstay approach for BED, pharmacological treatments, either alone or in combination with psychotherapy, can be an important option for adults. Not all patients have access to, a desire for, or a response to psychotherapy. To date, only lisdexamfetamine dimesylate (LDX), a stimulant originally indicated for attention-deficit/hyperactivity disorder (ADHD), has been approved by the U.S. Food and Drug Administration (FDA) for treating BED in adults. However, other classes of medications have shown efficacy in randomized trials and are commonly used off-label—especially when patients have symptoms of both BED and other diagnoses. The major pharmacological options, which include stimulants/anti-ADHD medications, antidepressants, anticonvulsants, and antiobesity agents, are discussed in the following subsections, and a recent comprehensive review, by McElroy (2017), is available. It is worth highlighting that BED patients often show high placebo response rates to pharmacological agents, which underscores the importance of conducting randomized, double-blind, controlled studies in this population. To date, there have been no medications trials for the treatment of BED in adolescents.

Stimulants and Other Anti–ADHD Medications

Initially a treatment for ADHD in children and adults, LDX became the first medication to receive an FDA indication for the treatment of moderate to severe BED. Its use is supported by several randomized studies (Level 1). For example, McElroy et al. (2015) compared 11 weeks of LDX (30 mg, 50 mg, or 70 mg) with placebo. Although LDX at the 30-mg dosage did not differ significantly from placebo, both of the higher dosages demonstrated significantly greater rates of 4-week abstinence from binge eating (abstinence rates: placebo, 21%; 30 mg, 35%; 50 mg, 42%; 70 mg, 50%). LDX is not indicated for weight loss, although patients taking the 50–70 mg dosages lost about 5 kg compared with 0.1 kg while receiving placebo. The most common side effects were dry mouth (36%), decreased appetite (21%), insomnia (13%), and headaches (12%). Patients with any Axis I disorder, including depression, were excluded from the trial. LDX carries a FDA boxed warning regarding risk of substance abuse and dependence and is contraindicated in patients with a prior history of stimulant abuse. Longer-term safety and efficacy of LDX as a maintenance BED treatment have been examined by Gasior et al. (2017), who reported on a 12-month open label extension study of the 50 mg and 70 mg dosages. Small but statistically significant increases in heart rate (an average of 6–7 beats per minute) and blood pressure were found, which could be a problem for some individuals with cardiovascular vulnerability. In another study, Hudson et al. (2017) investigated the risk of relapse in patients who had originally responded to an open-label 12-week trial of LDX and were subsequently randomly assigned either to continue with LDX or to receive placebo instead over a 26-week period. Relapse rates were significantly lower (3%) among those randomly assigned to continue LDX compared with those switched to placebo (32%). The authors noted that the safety and side effect profiles of longer-term LDX were similar to those found previously in ADHD trials and that the relapse rate was unexpectedly low among those randomly assigned to receive placebo.

Relatively few other stimulants or anti-ADHD medications have been tested with BED patients to date. Atomoxetine (Level 2), a nonstimulant norepinephrine reuptake inhibitor, showed superiority over placebo in a randomized trial (McElroy et al. 2007a), with abstinence from binge eating (no binge episodes in the last week of the 10-week trial) significantly greater (70%) among those taking atomoxetine than among those receiving placebo (32%). Weight losses were also greater, with atomoxetine associated with a 2.7-kg loss compared with 0.0 kg for placebo. Side effects were significantly greater with atomoxetine; these included dry mouth, nausea, nervousness, and insomnia.

The stimulant methylphenidate (Level 3) was compared with CBT for BED in a small pilot investigation (Quilty et al. 2015). No significant differences were found in effectiveness for binge eating after 12 weeks of treatment, but significant decreases in weight were found only for methylphenidate and not for CBT.

There are advantages and limitations when considering stimulants/anti-ADHD medications for BED. LDX has the advantage of being the only FDA-approved medication for moderate to severe BED, and trials show it to be an effective treatment for binge eating. LDX reportedly is well tolerated, although it can cause insomnia if administered after the early morning or in high dosages. Disadvantages for using stimulants in BED include the potential for abuse, which has led to a FDA boxed warning for LDX. Thus, LDX should not be used in patients with a history of drug or alcohol abuse. Because of its small but measurable effects on heart rate and blood pressure, LDX should be avoided in patients with cardiovascular disease. It is important to underscore that although LDX is associated with weight loss, it is not indicated for the treatment of obesity. It is also worth highlighting that trials of LDX to date specifically excluded those with comorbid depression or bipolar disorder. Because LDX was introduced fairly recently, more studies are needed to answer questions such as its use in children/adolescents and its efficacy in comparison to other medication options (e.g., other stimulants) and psychotherapy.

Antidepressant Medications

Antidepressants, including selective serotonin reuptake inhibitors (SSRIs; e.g., fluoxetine, sertraline, citalopram, fluvoxamine), serotonin-norepinephrine reuptake inhibitors (SNRIs; e.g., duloxetine, venlafaxine), bupropion, and tricyclics (e.g., desipramine), have shown efficacy in reducing binge eating in patients with BED, at least in the short run, though with little effect on weight loss. Of these, the greatest evidence exists for SSRIs (Level 1). Stefano et al. (2008), in a meta-analysis of antidepressants for BED, reported that the abstinence rate from six SSRI trials was 41% compared with 22% for placebo. Antidepressants did not significantly differ from placebo on weight loss and rates of discontinuation were similar in both. For patients with depressive symptoms, however, those who received antidepressants showed significantly greater improvements than with placebo (Stefano et al. 2008). The antidepressant bupropion (Level 3) also has shown efficacy in reducing binge eating and weight in open-label trials; however, in a small, randomized trial by White and Grilo (2013), binge-free abstinence rates on bupropion (42%) did not differ statistically from those of placebo (27%). Such results highlight the frequently reported finding that patients with BED often demonstrate high placebo responses. Also worth highlighting is the fact that most antidepressant trials, like the medication trials more generally, do not include long-term follow-up. In placebo substitution maintenance trials, symptom relapses usually occur within a few months after the antidepressants are stopped. Finally, it should be noted that antidepressant dosages used to treat BED tend to be at the high end of the recommended range.

There are advantages and disadvantages of using antidepressants for BED. Antidepressants, particularly the SSRIs, have good evidence for being effective at reducing binge eating compared with placebos, at least in the short term. These medications are generally well tolerated and also are effective in treating comorbid distress such as depression, anxiety, and obsessive-compulsive symptoms. However, antidepressants, with the exception of bupropion, have generally not shown efficacy for weight loss, and some may be associated with weight gain.

Anticonvulsant Medications

Medications within the anticonvulsant class have also shown efficacy in reducing binge eating in patients with BED. Of these, topiramate (Level 1) is the best studied. Unlike antidepressants, which in general are weight neutral or may promote weight gain, topiramate has been associated with weight loss and reductions in binge frequency at both posttreatment and follow-up (for review, see Arbaizar et al. 2008). For example, in the largest randomized trial of topiramate to date (McElroy et al. 2007b), binge days decreased from 4.6 to 0.9 per week among those taking topiramate for 16 weeks compared with decreases from 4.6 to 2.2 per week for those receiving placebo. One-week abstinence rates from binge eating were 58% for topiramate and 29% for placebo. In another study in which topiramate was continued for 42 weeks in an open-label extension after a 14-week randomized trial, reductions in binge eating and body weight were maintained (McElroy et al. 2004a). Most studies initiate topiramate at 25 mg, with target dosage ranges generally of 200–400 mg (Arbaizar et al. 2008). Importantly, rates of discontinuation due to side effects from topiramate can be high, and this limits the clinical utility of this medication. Common side effects include cognitive problems (e.g., memory and word finding difficulties), paresthesias, dry mouth, nausea, and somnolence. Also, patients with clinically significant comorbid depression were usually excluded in most studies.

The anticonvulsant zonisamide has been studied in both an open-label and randomized trials (e.g., McElroy et al. 2004b, 2006; Level 2). These studies showed that zonisamide, given at dosages of 100–600 mg/day, reduced binge eating and weight. An open-label study by Claudino et al. (2007) found that zonisamide (dosages 50–200 mg/day), when combined with CBT, led to significantly greater improvements in 7-day binge eating abstinence (84%) compared with CBT plus placebo (61%). Weight losses of more than 10% were also significantly greater in the CBT plus topiramate group (33%) compared with the CBT plus placebo group (11.5%). Patients who continued to receive zonisamide over a 1-year follow-up maintained these improvements. Side effects on zonisimide (e.g., altered taste, fatigue, dry mouth, and cognitive impairment), as with topiramate, have led to discontinuation.

There are advantages and disadvantages of anticonvulsants for BED. The anticonvulsants described here are generally effective at reducing binge eating and weight. Side effects, however, limit their tolerability for many patients.

Antiobesity Medications

The rationale for using antiobesity medications is based on the fact that many BED patients are overweight or obese, which increases their risk for obesity-related morbidity and mortality. To date, the antiobesity medications D-fenfluramine and sibutramine are no longer available because of associated serious adverse events, including pulmonary hypertension, heart valve defects, and stroke. Of the remaining antiobesity agents, the lipase inhibitor orlistat (Level 2) has the most data for efficacy (Golay et al. 2005; Grilo and Masheb 2007). For example, Golay et al. (2005) demonstrated that obese BED patients had significantly greater percentages of weight loss (7.4% vs. 2.3%) after randomization to 24 weeks of orlistat (120 mg three times per day) versus placebo, respectively. Both groups showed reduced rates of binge episodes/week (orlistat, 5.4 to 1; placebo, 6.2 to 1.7), and the likelihood of continuing to be diagnosed with BED did not differ by treatment condition at the end of the study (Golay et al. 2005). Interestingly, dropout rates were higher in the placebo group (29%) than in the orlistat group (11%), and the only patients who discontinued the study because of adverse events were from the group receiving placebo. In a study of 12 weeks of CBT–guided self-help with adjunctive orlistat versus CBT–guided self-help with placebo (Grilo et al. 2005), dropout rates were higher in those assigned to receive orlistat (8%) than in those receiving placebo (0%). Gastrointestinal side effects (e.g., oily stools) from orlistat were related to its mechanism of action. The CBT–guided self-help plus orlistat condition showed significantly greater rates of 28-day binge abstinence at post-treatment compared with the CBT–guided self-help plus placebo condition (64% vs. 36%), although this difference was not maintained at 3-month follow-up (52% in both). Weight losses of at least 5% were significantly greater in the CBT–guided self-help plus orlistat condition compared with the CBT–guided self-help plus placebo condition at both post-treatment (36% vs. 8%) and 3-month follow-up (32% vs. 8%).

Another antiobesity drug, phentermine (up to 30 mg/day), was tested in a small open trial ($n=16$) of overweight binge eaters (Level 3). The patients all received 20 sessions of CBT and up to 60 mg/day of fluoxetine (Devlin et al. 2000). Medication maintenance was available for up to 3 years. Reductions in binge eating, weight, and psychological symptoms (e.g., depression, eating psychopathology) were observed after the active phase of treatment, with 12 of the initial 16 (75%) subjects achieving 2-week binge abstinence. By 12-month follow-up, however, most of the weight initially lost had been regained, and by the end of follow-up there was no longer a significant difference in weight from baseline. Discontinuation rates from medications were high. By the 18-month follow-up, only two (12.5%) patients were still taking both phentermine and fluoxetine, with lack of efficacy cited as a primary reason for discontinuing phentermine.

Other FDA-approved antiobesity medications, such as bupropion-naltrexone, liraglutide, and phentermine-topiramate extended release, have limited data to date, making it difficult to assign a code. Robert et al. (2015) reported that individuals with subthreshold BED randomly assigned to receive liraglutide versus a diet-exercise control showed greater improvements in binge eating and weight loss relative to diet-exercise only. A post-hoc analysis of obese patients with depression who were given bupropion-naltrexone, of whom 91% reported binge-eating symptoms, reported significant reductions in binge eating, depression, and weight (Guerdjikova et al. 2017b); the dropout rate was 48%, with side effects (e.g., nausea, constipation, headache) being the most common reason. Guerdjikova et al. (2015) also reported a case series of two individuals with obesity and binge eating who experienced binge abstinence and weight loss with phentermine-topiramate extended release. A large, randomized, crossover trial of phentermine-topiramate extended release is under way (Dalai et al. 2018).

There are advantages and disadvantages to consider when using antiobesity medications for BED. These medications show preliminary efficacy in terms of binge eating and weight loss, although more investigations are needed. The findings to date suggest that side effects often limit their tolerability.

Other Medications

Other medications, such as naltrexone, ALKS-33 (a novel opiate antagonist), baclofen, and acamprosate, have been used to treat binge eating (Level 3). These drugs have been used to decrease cravings, such as with alcohol and opiates, which is part of the rationale for their use with binge eating. Whereas acamprosate (McElroy et al. 2011) and baclofen (Corwin et al. 2012) were superior to placebo for reducing binge eating and body weight, neither naltrexone (Alger et al. 1991) nor ALKS-33 (McElroy et al. 2013) separated from placebo.

Combined Medication and Psychotherapy Treatments

Relatively few studies have evaluated the potential added value of combining psychotherapy with medications when treating BED (for review, see Grilo et al. 2016). Overall, it appears that there is no additional benefit in terms of binge-related outcomes for combining an antidepressant with psychotherapy (e.g., CBT). Some studies, however, have shown that the addition of an antidepressant is associated with improvement in depressive symptoms. Furthermore, the addition of an antidepressant may enhance weight loss. In terms of the anticonvulsants, Claudino et al. (2007) in their study found that both binge-eating reduction and weight loss outcomes were greater when topiramate was added to CBT.

Because many of the newer BED pharmacological treatments such as LDX have not yet been tested in combination with psychotherapy, information is limited as to any potential benefits. More studies are needed, especially those that allow comparison of psychotherapy alone, medications alone, and combined medication with psychotherapy. In common practice medications are added to psychotherapy when patients show limited benefit from an initial trial of psychotherapy or when a comorbid disorder such as depression, anxiety, or obsessive-compulsive disorder is present.

Transcranial Magnetic Stimulation

Transcranial magnetic stimulation (TMS) is an experimental nonpharmacological approach to targeting BED symptoms. Burgess et al. (2016) investigated the effects of transcranial direct current stimulation (tDCS) on binge-eating frequency, binge-eating desire, food craving, and food intake in 30 adults with full or subthreshold BED (i.e., all criteria were met except for binge frequency per week). Participants received a 20-minute 2-milliampere session of tDCS targeting the dorsolateral prefrontal cortex (anode right/cathode left) and a "sham" session with participants blind to session type. In comparison with the sham session, tDCS significantly decreased food craving, food intake, and desire to binge eat on the day of administration but did not reduce binge-eating frequency. Although additional research is necessary, TMS may be a noninvasive treatment option for BED (Level 4).

Predictors and Moderators of Outcome

A variety of patient characteristics (e.g., age, sex, ethnicity/race, weight), psychiatric comorbidities, and eating behavior variables have been tested as predictors or moderators of treatment outcome. However, none of these variables have been reliably shown to predict or moderate treatment outcome (Grilo 2017). Conflicting data exist on the validity of BED specifiers and their use in predicting treatment outcome (Dakanalis et al. 2017; Gianini et al. 2017; Nakai et al. 2017; Smith et al. 2017b). That said, the presence of overvaluation of shape/

weight on self-worth appears to have prognostic significance in that studies show that BED patients with overvaluation of weight/shape have less improvement in symptoms across treatments (Grilo 2013). For example, remission rates were 29% in participants with overvaluation compared with 57% in participants without overvaluation (Grilo et al. 2012, 2013). Additionally, participants with overvaluation benefited less from medication than from CBT (Grilo et al. 2012). Rapid response to treatment (generally defined as a 65% or 70% or greater reduction in binge eating by week 4) also appears to have prognostic significance in that those with rapid response compared with nonrapid responders show greater likelihood of achieving remission after psychological and pharmacological interventions as well as of losing more weight in BWL treatments (Grilo 2017; Nazar et al. 2017).

Summary

There are a variety of effective interventions for BED. Current evidence points to CBT either in individual or in group format as a good first-line treatment for BED primarily because of the more substantial evidence base for this modality. IPT and DBT are reasonable alternative treatments. Various pharmacological treatments can be used, particularly LDX and anticonvulsants. We await additional evidence regarding whether experimental psychological treatments, such as VR/AR treatments, ABBT, involving the partner in treatment with UNITE, TMS, or other pharmacological treatments, are efficacious, with either added benefit or appropriateness for select individuals.

Prospective patients can be informed that CBT, IPT, and DBT have been found to effectively reduce binge eating but not weight, whereas BWL approaches have been found to effectively reduce weight but are less effective at reducing binge eating (Berkman et al. 2015; Peat et al. 2017). Individuals should be made aware of the likelihood for long-term weight regain following BWL intervention (McElroy et al. 2015). Because of evidence that binge abstinence is associated with weight loss, it should be emphasized that individuals desiring weight loss would ideally reduce their binge-eating behaviors prior to specific weight management attempts.

National Institute for Health and Care Excellence (2017) guidelines for the treatment of BED recommend a stepped-care approach in which interventions are provided sequentially according to response to treatment. Within this approach, patients start with the simplest, least intrusive, and least costly treatment, with more complex or intensive interventions administered to patients not responding to that level of care. As a first step, clinicians encourage patients to consider an evidence-based guided self-help program. Indications for guided self-help may include mild symptom severity, lack of psychiatric comorbidity, and/or logistical, travel, or access barriers to treatment (Vocks et al. 2010). Because of the paucity of stepped-care studies for BED, it is not fully clear how patients who do not respond to guided self-help or other first-line treatments should be treated. For example, choices include changing to another evidence-based psychotherapy treatment, adding a medication, moving to a more intensive treatment setting, or persisting with the same intervention for a longer period. Figure 4–1 is a decision tree rank ordering clinical interventions based on the evidence base to help guide practitioner's decisions about treatment. It should be noted that any decision should consider the evidence base as well as patient-specific factors (e.g., access to resources, comorbidity, patient preferences, clinician's psychosocial formulation).

First-Line Treatment

Individual or group psychotherapy, with the most evidence for CBT, including guided self-help CBT.

- If there are mild symptoms, no psychiatric comorbidity, or lack of access to in-person care, consider guided self-help CBT first.
- If there are moderate to severe symptoms (or failure of initial guided self-help), consider individual or group in-person CBT.

Second-Line Treatment/Alternative Treatment

If CBT is not effective or not available, it is unclear what the hierarchy is for other treatments, but the recommendation would be to select a psychotherapy treatment—based on the patient's clinical conceptualization—or a medication as follows:

- If the primary mechanism underlying binge eating is a deficit in interpersonal functioning, select IPT.

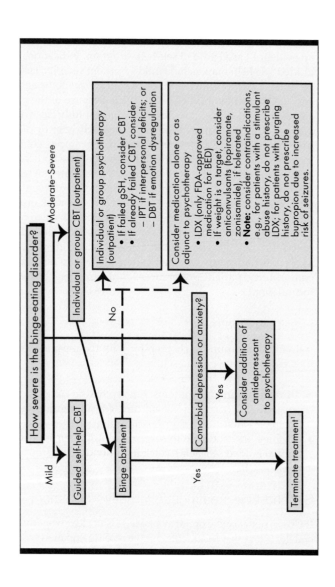

How severe is the binge-eating disorder?

Mild → Guided self-help CBT

Moderate–Severe → Individual or group CBT (outpatient)

Individual or group psychotherapy (outpatient)
- If failed gSH, consider CBT
- If already failed CBT, consider
  – IPT if interpersonal deficits; or
  – DBT if emotion dysregulation

Consider medication alone or as adjunct to psychotherapy
- LDX (only FDA-approved medication for BED)
- If weight is a target, consider anticonvulsants (topiramate, zonisamide), if tolerated
- **Note:** consider contraindications, e.g., for patients with a stimulant abuse history, do not prescribe LDX; for patients with purging history, do not prescribe bupropion due to increased risk of seizures.

No

Binge abstinent

Comorbid depression or anxiety?

Yes → Consider addition of antidepressant to psychotherapy

Yes → Terminate treatment[1]

FIGURE 4–1. (*opposite*) Decision tree rank ordering clinical interventions based on the evidence base to help guide practitioner's decisions about treatment.

Higher levels of care options are not included in the decision tree figure above due to the lack of evidence to support their prescription. However, if a patient fails multiple courses of outpatient psychotherapy or medication trials and exhibits severe binge-eating disorder (BED) symptoms or has serious physical complications, consider higher level of care options (e.g., partial hospitalization, inpatient).

[1]If the patient is binge abstinent but has significant weight-related concerns and/or complications due to overweight/obesity with desire for weight loss, consider weight loss approaches. Note, although psychotherapy does not tend to show weight losses on average, the evidence that the achievement of binge abstinence is associated with some weight loss, and that patients who binge eat are less like to respond to weight loss attempts, underscores the importance of targeting binge eating first before considering weight loss.

- If the primary mechanism underlying binge eating is a deficit in emotion regulation, select DBT.
- Medication alone or in combination with psychotherapy:
  - If there is presence of severe comorbid psychopathology (e.g., depression, anxiety, obsessive-compulsive disorder) and/or limited response to psychotherapy, consider selecting an antidepressant.
  - If no depression or anxiety present, select LDX (only FDA-approved medication for BED). If lack of response, consider an antidepressant, anticonvulsant (e.g., topiramate), and so forth.
  - If weight is a target, consider a medication that targets both binge eating and weight loss, such as an anticonvulsant (e.g., topiramate), if tolerated.
  - *Note:* Choices of medication also would be made based on the presence of contraindications. For example, patients who have abused stimulants would not be prescribed LDX, and patients with a history of purging behavior would not be prescribed bupropion due an increased risk of seizures.

Completed Course of Psychotherapy

- If the patient is binge abstinent, terminate treatment.
- If the patient is binge abstinent but has significant weight related concerns and/or complications due to overweight/

obesity with desire for weight loss, consider weight loss approaches. Since psychotherapy is not generally associated with weight loss, patients may want to initially focus on weight loss. Weight loss may be their primary concern. It is important to convey the value of targeting binge abstinence first, as the evidence shows that sustained binge abstinence is associated with some weight loss. Also, patients who continue to binge eat are less likely to respond to weight loss attempts.

Treatments Illustrated

Cognitive-Behavioral Therapy for Binge-Eating Disorder (see Case 1)

CBT (see Table 4–1) was chosen as the first-line treatment for Valerie because of the seemingly direct link between her negative evaluations of her weight and shape and her restrictive behaviors, which led to her binge eating. Following guidelines set for adults, either CBT or IPT could be considered for this type of presentation. Given the patient's endorsement of maladaptive thoughts about her weight and shape and increased worry about her health, which directly led to her restrictive behavior, the treating clinician believed that CBT would be indicated as a first-line treatment. If there had been a clear indicator that an interpersonal relationship or the patient's endorsement of her role in the family or athletic system was a maintaining factor for the binge behaviors, IPT could have been considered. In CBT for BED, treatment is split into stages, each with specific treatment targets. In the first stage of treatment, psychoeducation on the CBT model, eating disorders, and normalization of eating are primary targets. This stage also includes linking a tailored CBT conceptualization together with the client, one that outlines how her thoughts (cognitions) and feelings drive her binge behaviors. Specifically, this means working with the patient to demonstrate how the worry about her weight impacts her life and leads her to severe daytime restriction, intense frustration and strong hunger in the evenings, and subsequent out-of-control eating. She should also be educated about how the guilt and shame around her eating behaviors fuel her negative evaluation of her weight and shape, perpetuating the cycle. Collaboration with the patient to illustrate this feedback loop is an integral part of creating treatment goals. Of equal importance is the introduction and buy-in to the tools the patient will learn to use to break this maladaptive feedback loop, specifically self-monitoring, meal logging, and normalizing eating behaviors by eating three meals plus at least two snacks a day.

After a review in the second stage, the third stage's treatment targets include helping the patient identify triggers for bingeing as well as using stimulus control strategies and gradual exposure to feared foods and situations to prevent binge eating. In this case, the patient was bingeing on lower-calorie foods to avoid weight gain and was highly avoidant of foods not considered "healthy." Treatment includes carefully adding back feared foods into her diet in a systematic way. Additionally, in stage 3, specific maladaptive thoughts are addressed and targeted through cognitive restructuring; for example, the thought that the patient will not be accepted if she is not at her training weight leads to high anxiety and subsequent food restriction. Thus, the patient is taught how to evaluate evidence for and against her thoughts and develop a rational alternative way of thinking. This process includes using behavioral experiments to "test out" her thinking, for example, purposefully getting to and maintaining her training weight and observing how others around her respond. The patient is also taught alternative coping strategies for managing negative affect and anxiety about weight and eating, approaches such as progressive muscle relaxation, distraction, deep breathing, and seeking social support.

In stage 4, exposures are continued and the therapist and patient engage in problem solving around any obstacles that may be getting in the way of change. If there are interpersonal problems, these are addressed in this phase. For example, she learned how to effectively communicate with both her parents and her teammates and assertively set boundaries around comments regarding her eating habits and her weight. Reducing the number of comments she was hearing externally allowed her internal cognitive restructuring to become stronger and more believable. The final activity in stage 4 is a relapse prevention plan to recap treatment gains and address potential future obstacles and relapses before terminating treatment. In this case, it would be predicted that the patient would achieve binge abstinence and report a significant decrease in her distress by the end of treatment.

CBT and Medications (see Case 2)

The pattern of Samantha's eating led her to initiate psychotherapy with a therapist. Treatment followed a CBT model,

TABLE 4–1. General outline of treatment targets for enhanced cognitive-behavioral therapy

Stage 1

Engage in prospect of change and enhancing motivation to adhere to the treatment

Establish real-time self-monitoring via food and mood logs

Implement weekly weighing to expose the patient to fluctuations in weight and begin to decrease reactivity to weight and shape

Educate about and initiate a regular eating schedule

Stage 2

Review and revise formulation and continue to stabilize eating

Stage 3

Target

Overevaluation of shape and weight, body checking/ avoidance, "feeling fat"

Dietary restraint, problem solving, and binge analysis

Event- or mood-related changes in eating (including mood intolerance)

Undereating

Clinical perfectionism, core low self-esteem, and major interpersonal difficulties

Stage 4

Maintain changes and minimize relapse

Educate about relapse and mindsets

Detect problems early

Develop a maintenance plan

Discuss when to return/seek help

Termination

---

and there were substantial improvements: "I feel my relationship with food has improved substantially and the amount of time I spend thinking about food or my body has diminished somewhat." Her binge episodes became less frequent than when she began therapy about 6 months earlier (lowering from four or five times per week to about three times per week), but she still endorses feeling "stuck in the pattern," with her progress plateaued. Her mood remains down, and her therapist recommends that she seek consultation with a psychiatrist. She says she is interested in considering medications to try to get her binge eating and mood under better control. She wants to lose at least 15–20 lb (her current height is 5′4″ and her weight is 178 lb). She states her primary care doctor has recommended weight loss because Samantha is showing signs of prediabetes. Her therapist, however, cautions the patient from being overly focused on dieting.

Samantha's lack of a sufficient response in terms of binge-eating symptoms means that further treatment could be considered. One option would be to discuss with her the potential addition of IPT. Another option would be to add a medication, with the goal of enhancing not only her binge-eating outcomes but also improving her mood. Based on the data, an antidepressant, most likely an SSRI, would be a likely choice. Vyvanse would be less preferable in this situation given that it has not been approved for patients with comorbid depression. Bupropion would not be an option because it is contraindicated for patients with a current or prior diagnosis of bulimia nervosa or anorexia nervosa due to the higher incidence of seizures that has been noted in such patients.

The goal of the addition of an SSRI would be for the patient to achieve abstinence from binge eating and a reduction in her symptoms of depression and anxiety. Once those goals are achieved, the status of the patient's weight would be reevaluated. It is expected that binge-eating abstinence itself would result in some weight loss. However, if the patient's weight remains problematic from a medical standpoint, options include adding a medication focusing on the combination of continued binge abstinence and weight loss. Topiramate would be a logical choice, given the data supporting its efficacy with both, especially if the patient has not completely remitted from binge eating. At this point, Vvyanse is only indicated for patients with moderate to severe binge eating and, in addition, is not intended for use when the sole goal is weight loss given the risks (e.g., abuse) of using stimulants for weight control.

Common Outcomes and Complications

- Many individuals with BED have not had their disorder diagnosed or are untreated. Without treatment, they are likely to experience a chronic, fluctuating course of symptoms. If they are treated, a modest number will experience remission from symptoms, at least for up to 2 years (long-term follow-up studies are lacking).

- BED is associated with a higher rate of hospitalization, outpatient care, and emergency department visits as well as higher economic cost compared with healthy control subjects (Ágh et al. 2016; Ling et al. 2017). Annual direct and indirect healthcare costs are estimated at, on average, $20,194 and $19,000 per year, respectively.

- BED may result in medical issues (see "Common Comorbidities" earlier in this chapter). Women in midlife (40 years or older) with BED appear to have significantly more medical complications than women with BED in their young adult years (18–25) (Elran-Barak et al. 2015); specifically, one or more medical comorbidities were reported by 83% of midlife women with BED compared with 40% of young adults. The medical complications that arise from eating disorder symptoms could be intensified at midlife due to the body's diminished ability to resist and rebound from physical insult in older age or cumulative effects due to chronicity of illness (Fairburn and Harrison 2003).

- Among adolescents and young adults, binge eating has been found to predict future obesity, depression, and substance use (Sonneville et al. 2012).

- Suicide attempts may occur. Attempted suicide history is about five times more likely in individuals with BED compared with those without BED (Forrest et al. 2017). One study found that about 12.5% of adult (mean 39.5, SD 8.2 years) outpatients with BED had attempted suicide over their lifetime (Carano et al. 2012).

- In general, individuals with eating disorders are at increased risk of death secondary to complications from the disorder or to suicide, and older age has been associated with a relatively increased mortality rate (Arcelus et al. 2011). In a large sample of consecutively admitted inpatients followed through the German Civil Registry, the standardized mortality ratio of BED was 1.50 (Fichter and Quadflieg 2016). Lack of power has precluded meta-analytic studies to explore causal factors of fatal suicide attempts in BED samples (Smith et al. 2017a).

Resources and Further Reading

Training Resources

CBT—Oxford Cognitive Therapy Centre: https://www.octc.co.uk/
training
DBT—Behavioral Tech: https://behavioraltech.org/

Agras WS, Apple RF: Overcoming Eating Disorders: A Cognitive-
Behavioral Therapy Approach for Bulimia Nervosa and Binge-
Eating Disorder: Therapist Guide (Treatments That Work). New
York, Oxford University Press, 2007
Fairburn CG: Cognitive Behavioral Therapy and Eating Disorders.
New York, Guilford, 2008
Safer DL, Telch CF, Chen EY: Dialectical Behavior Therapy for Binge
Eating and Bulimia. New York, Guilford, 2009

Further Reading

Assessment/Diagnosis

Mitchell JE, Peterson CB: Assessment of Eating Disorders. New York,
Guilford, 2007

Treatment

Agras WS, Robinson A: The Oxford Handbook of Eating Disorders
(Oxford Library of Psychology), 2nd Edition. New York, Oxford
University Press, 2018
Apple RF, Agras SW: Overcoming Your Eating Disorder: A Cogni-
tive-Behavioral Therapy Approach for Bulimia Nervosa and
Binge-Eating Disorder Workbook (Treatments That Work). New
York, Oxford University Press, 2007
Craighead LW: The Appetite Awareness Workbook: How to Listen to
Your Body and Overcome Bingeing, Overeating, and Obsession
with Food. Oakland, CA, New Harbinger, 2006
Fairburn CG: Overcoming Binge Eating. New York, Guilford, 1995
Grilo CM, Mitchell JE: The Treatment of Eating Disorders: A Clinical
Handbook. New York, Guilford, 2011
Matz J, Frankel E: Beyond a Shadow of a Diet: The Comprehensive
Guide to Treating Binge Eating Disorder, Compulsive Eating, and
Emotional Overeating. New York, Routledge, 2014
Mitchell JE, Devlin MJ, de Zwaan M, et al: Binge-Eating Disorder:
Clinical Foundations and Treatment. New York, Guilford, 2007
Safer DL, Adler S, Masson PC: The DBT Solution for Emotional Eat-
ing: A Proven Program to Break the Cycle of Bingeing and Out-
of-Control Eating. New York, Guilford, 2017
Thompson-Brenner H: Casebook of Evidence-Based Therapy for Eat-
ing Disorders. New York, Guilford, 2015

References

Ágh T, Kovács G, Supina D, et al: A systematic review of the health-related quality of life and economic burdens of anorexia nervosa, bulimia nervosa, and binge eating disorder. Eat Weight Disord 21(3):353–364, 2016 26942768

Agras WS, Telch CF, et al: Weight-loss, cognitive-behavioral, and desipramine treatments in binge eating disorder: an additive design. Behav Ther 25(2):225–238, 1994

Alger SA, Schwalberg MD, Bigaouette JM, et al: Effect of a tricyclic antidepressant and opiate antagonist on binge-eating behavior in normoweight bulimic and obese, binge-eating subjects. Am J Clin Nutr 53(4):865–871, 1991 2008865

Ambrogne JA: Assessment, diagnosis, and treatment of binge eating disorder. J Psychosoc Nurs Ment Health Serv 55(8):32–38, 2017 28771285

Ansell EB, Grilo CM, White MA: Examining the interpersonal model of binge eating and loss of control over eating in women. Int J Eat Disord 45(1):43–50, 2012 21321985

American Psychiatric Association: Diagnostic and Statistical Manual of Mental Disorders, 4th Edition. Washington, DC, American Psychiatric Association, 1994

American Psychiatric Association: Diagnostic and Statistical Manual of Mental Disorders, 5th Edition. Arlington, VA, American Psychiatric Association, 2013

American Psychiatric Association: Feeding and Eating Disorders: DSM-5 Selections. Arlington, VA, American Psychiatric Publishing, 2015

Arbaizar B, Gómez-Acebo I, Llorca J: Efficacy of topiramate in bulimia nervosa and binge-eating disorder: a systematic review. Gen Hosp Psychiatry 30(5):471–475, 2008 18774432

Arcelus J, Mitchell AJ, Wales J, et al: Mortality rates in patients with anorexia nervosa and other eating disorders. A meta-analysis of 36 studies. Arch Gen Psychiatry 68(7):724–731, 2011 21727255

Arcelus J, Haslam M, Farrow C, et al: The role of interpersonal functioning in the maintenance of eating psychopathology: a systematic review and testable model. Clin Psychol Rev 33(1):156–167, 2013 23195616

Baker JH, Runfola CD: Eating disorders in midlife women: a perimenopausal eating disorder? Maturitas 85:112–116, 2016 26857889

Berkman ND, Brownley KA, Peat CM, et al: Management and Outcomes of Binge-Eating Disorder. Comparative Effectiveness Reviews, No 160. Rockville, MD, Agency for Healthcare Research and Quality, 2015

Blostein F, Assari S, Caldwell CH: Gender and ethnic differences in the association between body image dissatisfaction and binge eating disorder among blacks. J Racial Ethn Health Disparities 4(4):529–538, 2017 27352115

Bravender T, Bryant-Waugh R, Herzog D, et al: Classification of child and adolescent eating disturbances. Workgroup for Classification of Eating Disorders in Children and Adolescents (WCEDCA). Int J Eat Disord 40(suppl):S117–S122, 2007 17868122

Burgess EE, Sylvester MD, Morse KE, et al: Effects of transcranial direct current stimulation (tDCS) on binge eating disorder. Int J Eat Disord 49(10):930–936, 2016 27159906

Carano A, De Berardis D, Campanella D, et al: Alexithymia and suicide ideation in a sample of patients with binge eating disorder. J Psychiatr Pract 18(1):5–11, 2012 22261978

Cesa GL, Manzoni GM, Bacchetta M, et al: Virtual reality for enhancing the cognitive behavioral treatment of obesity with binge eating disorder: randomized controlled study with one-year follow-up. J Med Internet Res 15(6):e113, 2013 23759286

Citrome L: Binge-eating disorder and comorbid conditions: differential diagnosis and implications for treatment. J Clin Psychiatry 78(suppl 1):9–13, 2017 28125173

Claudino AM, de Oliveira IR, Appolinario JC, et al: Double-blind, randomized, placebo-controlled trial of topiramate plus cognitive-behavior therapy in binge-eating disorder. J Clin Psychiatry 68(9):1324–1332, 2007 17915969

Corwin RL, Boan J, Peters KF, et al: Baclofen reduces binge eating in a double-blind, placebo-controlled, crossover study. Behav Pharmacol 23(5–6):616–625, 2012 22854310

Culbert KM, Racine SE, Klump KL: Research review: what we have learned about the causes of eating disorders—a synthesis of sociocultural, psychological, and biological research. J Child Psychol Psychiatry 56(11):1141–1164, 2015 26095891

Dakanalis A, Colmegna F, Riva G, et al: Validity and utility of the DSM-5 severity specifier for binge-eating disorder. Int J Eat Disord 50(8):917–923, 2017 28245061

Dalai SS, Adler S, Najarian T, et al: Study protocol and rationale for a randomized double-blinded crossover trial of phentermine-topiramate ER versus placebo to treat binge eating disorder and bulimia nervosa. Contemp Clin Trials 64:173–178, 2018 29038069

de Zwaan M, Mitchell JE, Howell LM, et al: Characteristics of morbidly obese patients before gastric bypass surgery. Compr Psychiatry 44(5):428–434, 2003 14505305

Devlin MJ, Goldfein JA, Carino JS, et al: Open treatment of overweight binge eaters with phentermine and fluoxetine as an adjunct to cognitive-behavioral therapy. Int J Eat Disord 28(3):325–332, 2000 10942919

Elran-Barak R, Fitzsimmons-Craft EE, Benyamini Y, et al: Anorexia nervosa, bulimia nervosa, and binge eating disorder in midlife and beyond. J Nerv Ment Dis 203(8):583–590, 2015 26164423

Fairburn CG: Overcoming Binge Eating. New York, Guilford, 1995

Fairburn CG: Cognitive Behavioral Therapy and Eating Disorders. New York, Guilford, 2008

Fairburn CG, Harrison PJ: Eating disorders. Lancet 361(9355):407–416, 2003 12573387

Fairburn CG, Rothwell ER: Apps and eating disorders: a systematic clinical appraisal. Int J Eat Disord 48(7):1038–1046, 2015 25728705

Fairburn CG, Cooper Z, Shafran R: Enhanced cognitive behavior therapy for eating disorders ("CBT-E"): an overview, in Cognitive Behavioral Therapy and Eating Disorders. Edited by Fairburn CG. New York, Guilford, 2008, pp 23–34

Fandiño J, Moreira RO, Preissler C, et al: Impact of binge eating disorder in the psychopathological profile of obese women. Compr Psychiatry 51(2):110–114, 2010 20152289

Favaro A, Santonastaso P: Suicidality in eating disorders: clinical and psychological correlates. Acta Psychiatr Scand 95(6):508–514, 1997 9242846

Ferrer-García M, Gutiérrez-Maldonado J, Pla-Sanjuanelo J, et al: A randomised controlled comparison of second-level treatment approaches for treatment-resistant adults with bulimia nervosa and binge eating disorder: assessing the benefits of virtual reality cue exposure therapy. Eur Eat Disord Rev 25(6):479–490, 2017 28804985

Fichter MM, Quadflieg N: Mortality in eating disorders—results of a large prospective clinical longitudinal study. Int J Eat Disord 49(4):391–401, 2016 26767344

Forrest LN, Zuromski KL, Dodd DR, et al: Suicidality in adolescents and adults with binge-eating disorder: Results from the national comorbidity survey replication and adolescent supplement. Int J Eat Disord 50(1):40–49, 2017 27436659

Gasior M, Hudson J, Quintero J, et al: A phase 3, multicenter, open-label, 12-month extension safety and tolerability trial of lisdexamfetamine dimesylate in adults with binge eating disorder. J Clin Psychopharmacol 37(3):315–322, 2017 28383364

Gianini L, Roberto CA, Attia E, et al: Mild, moderate, meaningful? Examining the psychological and functioning correlates of DSM-5 eating disorder severity specifiers. Int J Eat Disord 50(8):906–916, 2017 28489323

Golay A, Laurent-Jaccard A, Habicht F, et al: Effect of orlistat in obese patients with binge eating disorder. Obes Res 13(10):1701–1708, 2005 16286517

Grenon R, Schwartze D, Hammond N, et al: Group psychotherapy for eating disorders: a meta-analysis. Int J Eat Disord 50(9):997–1013, 2017 28771758

Grilo CM: Why no cognitive body image feature such as overvaluation of shape/weight in the binge eating disorder diagnosis? Int J Eat Disord 46(3):208–211, 2013 23233198

Grilo CM: Psychological and behavioral treatments for binge-eating disorder. J Clin Psychiatry 78(suppl 1):20–24, 2017 28125175

Grilo CM, Masheb RM: Rapid response predicts binge eating and weight loss in binge eating disorder: findings from a controlled trial of orlistat with guided self-help cognitive behavioral therapy. Behav Res Ther 45(11):2537–2550, 2007 17659254

Grilo CM, Masheb RM, Salant SL: Cognitive behavioral therapy guided self-help and orlistat for the treatment of binge eating disorder: a randomized, double-blind, placebo-controlled trial. Biol Psychiatry 57(10):1193–201, 2005 15866560

Grilo CM, White MA, Masheb RM: DSM-IV psychiatric disorder comorbidity and its correlates in binge eating disorder. Int J Eat Disord 42(3):228–234, 2009 18951458

Grilo CM, Masheb RM, Wilson GT, et al: Cognitive-behavioral therapy, behavioral weight loss, and sequential treatment for obese patients with binge-eating disorder: a randomized controlled trial. J Consult Clin Psychol 79(5):675–685, 2011 21859185

Grilo CM, Masheb RM, Crosby RD: Predictors and moderators of response to cognitive behavioral therapy and medication for the treatment of binge eating disorder. J Consult Clin Psychol 80(5):897–906, 2012 22289130

Grilo CM, White MA, Gueorguieva R, et al: Predictive significance of the overvaluation of shape/weight in obese patients with binge eating disorder: findings from a randomized controlled trial with 12-month follow-up. Psychol Med 43(6):1335–1344, 2013 22967857

Grilo CM, Reas DL, Mitchell JE: Combining pharmacological and psychological treatments for binge eating disorder: current status, limitations, and future directions. Curr Psychiatry Rep 18(6):55, 2016 27086316

Guerdjikova AI, Fitch A, McElroy SL: Successful treatment of binge eating disorder with combination phentermine/topiramate extended release. Prim Care Companion CNS Disord Apr 2, 17(2), 2015 26445680

Guerdjikova AI, Mori N, Casuto LS, McElroy SL: Binge eating disorder. Psychiatr Clin North Am 40(2):255–266, 2017a 28477651

Guerdjikova AI, Walsh B, Shan K, et al: Concurrent improvement in both binge eating and depressive symptoms with naltrexone/bupropion therapy in overweight or obese subjects with major depressive disorder in an open-label, uncontrolled study. Adv Ther 34(10):2307–2315, 2017b 28918581

Hildebrandt T, Michaelides A, Mackinnon D, et al: Randomized controlled trial comparing smartphone assisted versus traditional guided self-help for adults with binge eating. Int J Eat Disord 50(11):1313–1322, 2017 28960384

Hudson JI, Lalonde JK, Berry JM, et al: Binge-eating disorder as a distinct familial phenotype in obese individuals. Arch Gen Psychiatry 63(3):313–319, 2006 16520437

Hudson JI, Hiripi E, Pope HG Jr, et al: The prevalence and correlates of eating disorders in the National Comorbidity Survey Replication. Biol Psychiatry 61(3):348–358, 2007 16815322

Hudson JI, Lalonde JK, Coit CE, et al: Longitudinal study of the diagnosis of components of the metabolic syndrome in individuals with binge-eating disorder. Am J Clin Nutr 91(6):1568–1573, 2010 20427731

Hudson JI, McElroy SL, Ferreira-Cornwell MC, et al: Efficacy of lisdexamfetamine in adults with moderate to severe binge-eating disorder: a randomized clinical trial. JAMA Psychiatry 74(9):903–910, 2017 28700805

Javaras KN, Laird NM, Reichborn-Kjennerud T, et al: Familiality and heritability of binge eating disorder: results of a case-control family study and a twin study. Int J Eat Disord 41(2):174–179, 2008 18095307

Jones M, Luce KH, Osborne MI, et al: Randomized, controlled trial of an internet-facilitated intervention for reducing binge eating and over-weight in adolescents. Pediatrics 121(3):453–462, 2008 18310192

Juarascio AS, Manasse SM, Espel HM, et al: A pilot study of an acceptance-based behavioral treatment for binge eating disorder. J Contextual Behav Sci 6(1):1–7, 2017 28966910

Kessler RC, Berglund PA, Chiu WT, et al: The prevalence and correlates of binge eating disorder in the World Health Organization World Mental Health Surveys. Biol Psychiatry 73(9):904–914, 2013 23290497

Klump KL: Puberty as a critical risk period for eating disorders: a review of human and animal studies. Horm Behav 64(2):399–410, 2013 23998681

Kornstein SG: Epidemiology and recognition of binge-eating disorder in psychiatry and primary care. J Clin Psychiatry 78(suppl 1):3–8, 2017 28125172

Kristeller JL, Hallett CB: An exploratory study of a meditation-based intervention for binge eating disorder. J Health Psychol 4(3):357–363, 1999 22021603

Ling YL, Rascati KL, Pawaskar M: Dairect and indirect costs among patients with binge-eating disorder in the United States. Int J Eat Disord 50(5):523–532, 2017 27862132

Maldonado JG, Ferrer-Garcia M, Dakanalis A, et al: Virtual reality: applications to eating disorders, in The Oxford Handbook of Eating Disorders, 2nd Edition. Edited by Agras WS, Robinson A. New York, Oxford University Press, 2018, pp 470–491

Manzoni GM, Cesa GL, Bacchetta M, et al: Virtual reality–enhanced cognitive-behavioral therapy for morbid obesity: a randomized controlled study with 1 year follow-up. Cyberpsychol Behav Soc Netw 19(2):134–140, 2016 26430819

Marco JH, Perpiñá C, Botella C: Effectiveness of cognitive behavioral therapy supported by virtual reality in the treatment of body image in eating disorders: one year follow-up. Psychiatry Res 209(3):619–625, 2013 23499231

Marcus MD: Adapting treatment for patients with binge-eating disorder, in Handbook of Treatment for Eating Disorders. Edited by Garner DM, Garfinkel PR. New York, Guilford, 1997, pp 484–493

Marcus MD, Kalarchian MA: Binge eating in children and adolescents. Int J Eat Disord 34(suppl):S47–S57, 2003 12900986

Marcus MD, Wing RR, Fairburn CG: Cognitive behavioral treatment of binge eating vs. behavioral weight control on the treatment of binge eating disorder. Ann Behav Med 17:S090, 1995

Masheb RM, Grilo CM: Emotional overeating and its associations with eating disorder psychopathology among overweight patients with binge eating disorder. Int J Eat Disord 39(2):141–146, 2006 16231349

Masson PC, von Ranson KM, Wallace LM, et al: A randomized waitlist controlled pilot study of dialectical behaviour therapy guided self-help for binge eating disorder. Behav Res Ther 51(11):723–728, 2013 24029304

McElroy SL: Pharmacologic treatments for binge-eating disorder. J Clin Psychiatry 78(suppl 1):14–19, 2017 28125174

McElroy SL, Shapira NA, Arnold LM, et al: Topiramate in the long-term treatment of binge-eating disorder associated with obesity. J Clin Psychiatry 65(11):1463–1469, 2004a 15554757

McElroy SL, Kotwal R, Hudson JI, et al: Zonisamide in the treatment of binge-eating disorder: an open-label, prospective trial. J Clin Psychiatry 65(1):50–56, 2004b 14744168

McElroy SL, Kotwal R, Guerdjikova AI, et al: Zonisamide in the treatment of binge eating disorder with obesity: a randomized controlled trial. J Clin Psychiatry 67(12):1897–1906, 2006 17194267

McElroy SL, Guerdjikova A, Kotwal R, et al: Atomoxetine in the treatment of binge-eating disorder: a randomized placebo-controlled trial. J Clin Psychiatry 68(3):390–398, 2007a 17388708

McElroy SL, Hudson JI, Capece JA, et al: Topiramate for the treatment of binge eating disorder associated with obesity: a placebo-controlled study. Biol Psychiatry 61(9):1039–1048, 2007b 17258690

McElroy SL, Guerdjikova AI, Winstanley EL, et al: Acamprosate in the treatment of binge eating disorder: a placebo-controlled trial. Int J Eat Disord 44(1):81–90, 2011 21080416

McElroy SL, Guerdjikova AI, Blom TJ, et al: A placebo-controlled pilot study of the novel opioid receptor antagonist ALKS-33 in binge eating disorder. Int J Eat Disord 46(3):239–245, 2013 23381803

McElroy SL, Guerdjikova AI, Mori N, et al: Overview of the treatment of binge eating disorder. CNS Spectr 20(6):546–556, 2015 26594849

Milos G, Spindler A, Hepp U, et al: Suicide attempts and suicidal ideation: links with psychiatric comorbidity in eating disorder subjects. Gen Hosp Psychiatry 26(2):129–135, 2004 15038930

Mitchell JE: Medical comorbidity and medical complications associated with binge-eating disorder. Int J Eat Disord 49(3):319–323, 2016 26311499

Mitchell KS, Neale MC, Bulik CM, et al: Binge eating disorder: a symptom-level investigation of genetic and environmental influences on liability. Psychol Med 40(11):1899–1906, 2010 20132584

Binge-Eating Disorder　　　　　　　　　　　　　　　　　**145**

Nakai Y, Nin K, Noma S, et al: The impact of DSM-5 on the diagnosis and severity indicator of eating disorders in a treatment-seeking sample. Int J Eat Disord 50(11):1247–1254, 2017 28857236

National Institute for Health and Care Excellence: Eating Disorders: Recognition and Treatment (NG69). London, National Institute for Health and Care Excellence, May 2017. Available at: https://www.nice.org.uk/guidance/ng69. Accessed November 1, 2017.

Nazar BP, Gregor LK, Albano G, et al: Early response to treatment in eating disorders: a systematic review and a diagnostic test accuracy meta-analysis. Eur Eat Disord Rev 25(2):67–79, 2017 27928853

Niego SH, Kofman MD, Weiss JJ, et al: Binge eating in the bariatric surgery population: a review of the literature. Int J Eat Disord 40(4):349–359, 2007 17304586

Olguin P, Fuentes M, Gabler G, et al: Medical comorbidity of binge eating disorder. Eat Weight Disord 22(1):13–26, 2017 27553016

Palmisano GL, Innamorati M, Vanderlinden J: Life adverse experiences in relation with obesity and binge eating disorder: a systematic review. J Behav Addict 5(1):11–31, 2016 28092189

Pawaskar M, Witt EA, Supina D, et al: Impact of binge eating disorder on functional impairment and work productivity in an adult community sample in the United States. Int J Clin Pract 71(7):e12970, 2017 28741812

Peat CM, Berkman ND, Lohr KN, et al: Comparative effectiveness of treatments for binge-eating disorder: systematic review and network meta-analysis. Eur Eat Disord Rev 25(5):317–328, 2017 28467032

Peebles R, Wilson JL, Lock JD: How do children with eating disorders differ from adolescents with eating disorders at initial evaluation? J Adolesc Health 39(6):800–805, 2006 17116508

Pendleton VR, Goodrick GK, Poston WS, et al: Exercise augments the effects of cognitive-behavioral therapy in the treatment of binge eating. Int J Eat Disord 31(2):172–184, 2002 11920978

Perpiñá C, Marco JH, Botella C, et al: Tratamiento de la imagen corporal en los trastornos alimentarios mediante tratamiento cognitivo-comportamental apoyado con realidad virtual: resultados al año de seguimiento. Psicol Conductual 12:519–537, 2004

Quilty LC, Knyahnytska Y, Davis C, et al: Psychostimulant Medication in the Treatment of Binge-Eating Disorder: A Pilot Investigation. Paper presented at the annual meeting of the Society for Biological Psychiatry, Toronto, Ontario, Canada, May 2015

Ricca V, Castellini G, Lo Sauro C, et al: Correlations between binge eating and emotional eating in a sample of overweight subjects. Appetite 53(3):418–421, 2009 19619594

Rieger E, Van Buren DJ, Bishop M, et al: An eating disorder-specific model of interpersonal psychotherapy (IPT-ED): causal pathways and treatment implications. Clin Psychol Rev 30(4):400–410, 2010 20227151

Riener R, Schindler K, Ludvik B: Psychosocial variables, eating behavior, depression, and binge eating in morbidly obese subjects. Eat Behav 7(4):309–314, 2006 17056406

Riva G, Bacchetta M, Cesa G, et al: Six-month follow-up of inpatient experiential cognitive therapy for binge eating disorders. Cyberpsychol Behav 6(3):251–258, 2003 12855080

Riva G, Bacchetta M, Cesa G, et al: The use of VR in the treatment of eating disorders. Stud Health Technol Inform 99:121–163, 2004 15295149

Robert SA, Rohana AG, Shah SA, et al: Improvement in binge eating in non-diabetic obese individuals after 3 months of treatment with liraglutide: a pilot study. Obes Res Clin Pract 9(3):301–304, 2015 25870084

Ruffault A, Carette C, Lurbe I Puerto K, et al: Randomized controlled trial of a 12-month computerized mindfulness-based intervention for obese patients with binge eating disorder: the MindOb study protocol. Contemp Clin Trials 49:126–133, 2016 27370231

Runfola CD, Kirby JS, Baucom B, et al: Pilot study of a novel couple-based intervention for binge-eating disorder: UNITE. Paper presented at the International Conference on Eating Disorders, San Francisco, CA, May 2016

Safer DL, Couturier JL, Lock J: Dialectical behavior therapy modified for adolescent binge eating disorder: a case report. Cogn Behav Pract 14(2):157–167, 2007

Safer DC, Telch CF, Chen EY: Dialectical Behavior Therapy for Binge Eating and Bulimia. New York, Guilford, 2009

Safer DL, Robinson AH, Jo B: Outcome from a randomized controlled trial of group therapy for binge eating disorder: comparing dialectical behavior therapy adapted for binge eating to an active comparison group therapy. Behav Ther 41(1):106–120, 2010 20171332

Silverman W, Hinshaw S: The second special issue on evidence-based psychosocial treatments for children and adolescents: a 10-year update. J Clin Child Adolesc Psychol 37(1):1–7, 2008

Slevec JH, Tiggemann M: Predictors of body dissatisfaction and disordered eating in middle-aged women. Clin Psychol Rev 31(4):515–524, 2011 21239098

Smith AR, Zuromski KL, Dodd DR: Eating disorders and suicidality: what we know, what we don't know, and suggestions for future research. Curr Opin Psychol 22:63–67, 2017a 28846874

Smith KE, Ellison JM, Crosby RD, et al: The validity of DSM-5 severity specifiers for anorexia nervosa, bulimia nervosa, and binge-eating disorder. Int J Eat Disord 50(9):1109–1113, 2017b 28623853

Sonneville KR, Calzo JP, Horton NJ, et al: Body satisfaction, weight gain and binge eating among overweight adolescent girls. Int J Obes 36(7):944–949, 2012 22565419

Specker S, de Zwaan M, Raymond N, et al: Psychopathology in subgroups of obese women with and without binge eating disorder. Compr Psychiatry 35(3):185–190, 1994 8045108

Stefano SC, Bacaltchuk J, Blay SL, et al: Antidepressants in short-term treatment of binge eating disorder: systematic review and meta-analysis. Eat Behav 9(2):129–136, 2008 18329590

Stunkard AJ: Eating patterns and obesity. Psychiatr Q 33:284–295, 1959 13835451

Swanson SA, Crow SJ, Le Grange D, et al: Prevalence and correlates of eating disorders in adolescents. Results from the national co-morbidity survey replication adolescent supplement. Arch Gen Psychiatry 68(7):714–723, 2011 21383252

Tanofsky-Kraff M, Wilfley DE, Young JF, et al: A pilot study of inter-personal psychotherapy for preventing excess weight gain in ad-olescent girls at-risk for obesity. Int J Eat Disord 43(8):701–706, 2010 19882739

Tanofsky-Kraff M, Shomaker LB, Olsen C, et al: A prospective study of pediatric loss of control eating and psychological outcomes. J Abnorm Psychol 120(1):108–118, 2011 21114355

Telch CF, Agras WS, Linehan MM, et al: Group dialectical behavior therapy for binge-eating disorder: a preliminary, uncontrolled trial. Behav Ther 31(3):569–582, 2000

Telch CF, Agras WS, Linehan MM: Dialectical behavior therapy for binge eating disorder. J Consult Clin Psychol 69(6):1061–1065, 2001 11777110

Thornton LM, Watson HJ, Jangmo A, et al: Binge-eating disorder in the Swedish national registers: somatic comorbidity. Int J Eat Dis-ord 50(1):58–65, 2017 27642179

Urquhart CS, Mihalynuk TV: Disordered eating in women: implica-tions for the obesity pandemic. Can J Diet Pract Res 72(1):e115–e125, 2011 21382233

Vocks S, Tuschen-Caffier B, Pietrowsky R, et al: Meta-analysis of the effectiveness of psychological and pharmacological treatments for binge eating disorder. Int J Eat Disord 43(3):205–217, 2010 19402028

Wagner B, Nagl M, Dölemeyer R, et al: Randomized controlled trial of an internet-based cognitive-behavioral treatment program for binge-eating disorder. Behav Ther 47(4):500–514, 2016 27423166

White MA, Grilo CM: Bupropion for overweight women with binge-eating disorder: a randomized, double-blind, placebo-controlled trial. J Clin Psychiatry 74(4):400–406, 2013 23656848

Wilfley DE, Agras WS, Telch CF, et al: Group cognitive-behavioral therapy and group interpersonal psychotherapy for the nonpurg-ing bulimic individual: a controlled comparison. J Consult Clin Psychol 61(2):296–305, 1993 8473584

Wilfley DE, Welch RR, Stein RI, et al: A randomized comparison of group cognitive-behavioral therapy and group interpersonal psychotherapy for the treatment of overweight individuals with binge-eating disorder. Arch Gen Psychiatry 59(8):713–721, 2002 12150647

Wilfley DE, Citrome L, Herman BK: Characteristics of binge eating disorder in relation to diagnostic criteria. Neuropsychiatr Dis Treat 12:2213–2223, 2016 27621631

Wilson GT, Shafran R: Eating disorders guidelines from NICE. Lancet 365(9453):79–81, 2005 15639682

Wilson GT, Vitousek KM, Loeb KL: Stepped care treatment for eating disorders. J Consult Clin Psychol 68(4):564–572, 2000 10965631

Wilson GT, Wilfley DE, Agras WS, et al: Psychological treatments of binge eating disorder. Arch Gen Psychiatry 67(1):94–101, 2010 20048227

Wing RR, Hamman RF, Bray GA, et al: Achieving weight and activity goals among diabetes prevention program lifestyle participants. Obes Res 12(9):1426–1434, 2004 15483207

Yager J, Devlin MJ, Halmi KA, et al: Guideline Watch: Practice Guideline for the Treatment of Patients with Eating Disorders, 3rd Edition. Washington, DC, American Psychiatric Association, August 2012

Chapter 5

Avoidant/Restrictive Food Intake Disorder

Kathleen Kara Fitzpatrick, Ph.D.

Introduction

Avoidant/restrictive food intake disorder (ARFID) was introduced in DSM-5 (American Psychiatric Association 2013). Evaluation of patient characteristics found in the eating disorder not otherwise specified (EDNOS) category of DSM-IV-TR (American Psychiatric Association 2000) revealed a cluster of cases in which the individuals had symptoms that might be considered restrictive eating but without co-occurring body image distress (Bryant-Waugh and Nicholls 2011). Furthermore, these cases were often atypical from anorexia nervosa (AN) and bulimia nervosa (BN) in other ways, such as the increased prevalence of males, a younger age at presentation, and the trend toward low weight, but often without the frank starvation associated with AN (Bryant-Waugh et al. 2010; Turner and Bryant-Waugh 2004). Developmentally, ARFID made sense, as it simply expanded and refined the criteria for feeding disorder of infancy and early childhood (Bryant-Waugh et al. 2010). Clinically, treatment teams noted that individuals diagnosed in childhood with feeding disorder of infancy and early childhood were being moved into eating disorder treatment programs where they were often a "poor fit." ARFID diagnoses do not appear to predict a movement toward the more classic restrictive eating disorders (Bryant-Waugh and Kreipe 2012).

Although dietary restriction is a key feature of ARFID, the rejection of foods is driven more by specific fears around the food itself instead of unwanted side effects of eating, such as weight gain or growth, distinguishing it from the classic eating disorders. This results in foods being avoided based on the smell, taste, temperature, and/or appearance. In some cases, the rejection of foods can have a more acute onset, such as after a food-related trauma. Common examples include significant and sustained dietary restriction after choking or vomiting episodes or illness.

The key feature of ARFID is a persistent failure to take in a sufficient range of food to meet nutritional and energy needs. This includes patients presenting with low weight and without concurrent body image disturbance as well as normal-weight patients who get their caloric but not their nutritional needs met. Other children present with a simple disinterest in food, easily missing snacks and mealtimes or failing to fill up sufficiently, colloquially known as "eating like a bird," and maintaining a healthy weight only through strong parental efforts. This is sometimes referred to as a *disorder of homeostatic appetite*, referring to the failure to respond to their increased dietary needs with activity or through monitoring and responding to hunger. The focus on nutritional deficiency rather than specific weight criteria helps prevent diagnostic confusion with AN when a child with ARFID presents with low weight. There are no specific criteria for defining "nutritional deficiency," a term that has been broadly applied in clinical practice. Laboratory results and anecdotal clinical findings (e.g., anemia, zinc deficiency) have been used to support the diagnosis. Diagnosis can also be supported in the presence of a significantly limited dietary intake, as seen in extremely picky eaters.

Children with idiopathic gastrointestinal concerns and faltering weight, classically considered "failure to thrive," may be captured by ARFID criteria. In fact, one criterion focuses on enteral feed dependency and oral supplementation. Patients who are referred from other medical specialty clinics, most notably gastroenterology but also pain and endocrinology, may be appropriate for this diagnosis if it is determined that poor feeding and eating habits are underlying the symptom presentation. In one study, 50% of patients were referred from a medical clinic and 4% had significant allergies (Fisher et al. 2014). In Boston, 1.5% of a pediatric gastrointestinal population was found to have symptoms that met criteria for ARFID in a retrospective case review (Eddy et al. 2015). Higher prevalence rates of neurodevelopmental and developmental disabilities also occur in an ARFID population (Nicely et al. 2014; Thomas et al. 2017).

The development of the ARFID category helped create diagnostic clarification but also stimulated renewed research and clinical interest in these patients (Thomas et al. 2017).

Retrospective case review applying ARFID criteria suggests that ARFID makes up approximately 30% of the cases that had previously fallen under EDNOS (Pinhas et al. 2017). There remains concern that the ARFID category may unfairly pathologize more normative picky eaters or create anxiety among parents regarding their children's eating habits (Cardona Cano et al. 2015). It is worth repeating that ARFID symptoms must be enduring, extreme, and impairing, characteristics that are not typical of most childhood presentations of attenuated eating.

Key Diagnostic Checklist

❏ Symptoms

- Significant ongoing difficulty with feeding/eating behaviors that results in one of the following:

    - Failure to make appropriate weight gain or significant weight loss

    - Inability to meet nutritional needs, resulting in nutritional deficiency

    - Nutritional or energy needs can only be met with use of oral nutritional supplements or enteral feeds

    - Feeding/eating behaviors that result in significant impairment in psychosocial functioning

❏ No body image disturbance

❏ No current anorexia nervosa/bulimia nervosa

❏ Not due to a medical illness, cultural practice, or lack of available nutrition

Diagnostic Rule Outs

Medical

Medical rule outs are particularly important, because these can mask or exacerbate ARFID symptoms. Importantly, malnourishment can, itself, cause significant medical sequelae such as bradycardia, orthostasis, and electrolyte imbalances.

In severe cases of malnourishment, patients with ARFID should be monitored for refeeding syndrome before renourishment efforts take place.

- *Gastrointestinal disorders.* Gastrointestinal rule outs include all malabsorptive disorders and the inflammatory bowel disorders, which may influence nutritional status and also increase pain and nausea in idiosyncratic patterns. Issues such as chronic constipation and an impacted colon can also reduce intake and cause cramping and pain associated with eating.

- *Endocrine dysfunction.* Endocrine dysfunction should also be assessed to rule out issues related to growth (e.g., thyroid disease, pituitary insufficiency).

- *Food allergies.* Food allergies can cause dietary restriction, often through secondary pain, as well as through an elimination diet.

- *Pain.* Diffuse or idiopathic pain associated with eating can result from a range of factors (e.g., dental caries, mouth sores, esophageal strictures, superior mesenteric artery syndrome), and care should be taken to rule out medical issues related to pain.

Psychiatric

Psychiatric rule outs for ARFID fall largely within the category of eating disorders but also come from the following:

- *Anorexia nervosa.* AN is a critical rule out when thinking about ARFID; the key difference is in body image/dissatisfaction; ARFID is not associated with body image concerns, although both may have severely restricted intake, limited dietary range, and weight loss.

- *Major depressive disorder (MDD).* MDD can be associated with changes in appetite and eating that may appear to be similar to ARFID. This can be distinguished from ARFID as it occurs in the context of sad, down, low mood or irritability as well as associated symptoms. Both disorders can be diagnosed when symptoms are of sufficient number, intensity, and duration and are beyond what is expected in major depressive disorder.

- *Generalized anxiety disorder (GAD).* GAD is characterized by intense, frequent worry about a variety of topics, which also can cause headaches and stomachaches. In some cases, this can also cause appetite attenuation or nausea.

If worries are broad, and not just around food or intake, GAD may need to be ruled out. Both disorders can be diagnosed when symptoms are of sufficient number, intensity, and duration and are beyond what is expected in GAD.

- *Obsessive-compulsive disorder (OCD).* OCD can cause the individual to reject foods due to fears of contamination or based on concerns regarding the presentation and preparation of foods. On the surface this may appear to be ARFID, as the reason behind food rejection is based on sensory characteristics of the food. ARFID is not characterized by intrusive, distressing thoughts, or compulsive acts to reduce anxiety. There can be overlap between these disorders and as such, careful evaluations of both are important. Both disorders can be diagnosed when symptoms are of sufficient number, intensity, and duration and are beyond what is expected in obsessive-compulsive disorder.

- *Autism spectrum disorder (ASD).* Symptoms of ASD may overlap with ARFID, such as when there are rigidities around where, when, and how food might be consumed. These disorders may be characterized by rigid and heavily proscribed behaviors, although with ARFID this is around food preferences, where this is a much broader characterization of difficulties in those with autism spectrum disorders and other developmental delays. ARFID can be diagnosed when symptoms are of sufficient number, intensity, and duration and are beyond what is expected in autism.

Epidemiology and Risk Factors

Incidence/Prevalence

- Incidence and prevalence rates in population studies are unknown.
- ARFID appears to make up 2%–5% of the eating disorder population.
- ARFID can be diagnosed across the lifespan.
- ARFID is more commonly diagnosed in younger patients
- Typical age at onset is around 10–12 years.

Risks

- Little is known about cultural expression of eating symptoms in ARFID. It has been hypothesized that symptom expression might be different across different cultures and groups, but there is no evidence to support this.

- A Japanese study of an eating disorder population found that 11% had symptoms that met criteria for ARFID.
- Australian studies found that 0.3% of an eating disorder population had symptoms that met criteria for ARFID.
- Cultural eating practices or dietary restrictions should not be considered part of ARFID symptomatology.
- Little is known about risk factors and epidemiological factors for ARFID.
- At younger ages, ARFID appears to be diagnosed more in males.
- Traumatic episodes with food, including choking, vomiting, and illness, may increase risk for developing symptoms. For children who have had disruptions in normotypical eating, such as children requiring craniofacial surgery or those requiring tube feeds, specific retraining in eating behaviors may need to occur. This increases sensory sensitivities, and there is evidence to suggest that children who have been receiving enteral feeds likely require a very specific transition program to eat solid foods.
- In those cases of chronic failure to thrive post oral-facial/ maxillary surgeries or malformations or periods when a child was dependent on enteral or parenteral feeds and needs to "learn to eat again," there may be more layered and nuanced expectations around the role toward a mental health from physical health challenge.

Common Comorbidities

Psychiatric comorbidities with ARFID were evaluated in DSM-5 field trials and supported by follow-up evaluations. In general, these suggest that the main psychiatric comorbidities come from the anxiety disorders, attention disorders, and developmental disorders.

- Anxiety disorders, in particular GAD

  - High levels of anxiety are often seen in ARFID, and these psychiatric comorbidities can both predate as well as co-occur with ARFID. In a study by Thomas et al. (2017) the authors proposed that a subset of patients diagnosed with ARFID present with primary negative valence emotions (negative affect). Individuals coming from this proposed subset have heightened concerns about negative consequences (Thomas et al. 2017).

- Obsessive-compulsive disorder

- Specific phobias (common comorbid conditions all overlap with ARFID).

- Autism spectrum disorder (autism/developmental disorders)

Clinical Presentations

Jonathan—Extreme Picky Eater

Jonathan (Jo) presented at the outpatient eating disorders clinic for an intake at age 10. He was accompanied by his mother, who came ready with a binder to describe their **long history of "food battles" and the fact that he "just doesn't eat anything!"** According to Jo's mother, he was born at a healthy weight following a healthy, typical pregnancy. He was a bit of a fussy eater, with some gastroesophageal reflux disease in the first 6 months while breastfeeding, but when the family switched to soy formula these challenges disappeared. When Jo was introduced to solid foods, Jo's mother described him as "really slow to pick up on it" and reported that he would often gag and change his food preferences. They had fairly little trouble introducing fruits, but rice cereals and vegetables were often rejected quickly and difficult to establish.

Despite her concerns, however, Jo grew normally and the family was encouraged to relax and continue their efforts to feed him. Concerns were relatively stable until Jo went to school at age 5. He would often cry at snack time, and kindergarten teachers reported he would say he was not hungry, would skip a class-offered snack, and be clearly hungry and irritable toward lunch. However, at other times he would eat large portions of whatever was served. Teachers were concerned Jo was not getting enough to eat at home and asked his mother to provide snacks for him. This began a pattern of Jo's mother "packing meals, making sure he had what he needed for any trip where he might get hungry."

At the time they presented to the eating disorder clinic, Jo had developed a **strong preference for soft or crunchy foods** and enjoyed most carbohydrates and some fruits. He would **reject all vegetables, foods that he described as** "sticky" (e.g., honey, peanut butter), and most meats. He also **rejected mixed foods,** with the exception of pizza. However, even within this, Jo had **very strict preferences.** He only really ate a sufficient portion of pizza from his local pizzeria and only wanted mild cheddar cheese sticks from a particular grocery store, and he had **strong preferences about the ways foods were prepared,** according to his mother. For example, if a bagel was slightly overtoasted for his preference, he would not eat it and often would just skip breakfast. He would often complain that the foods packed in his lunch were too soggy, too cold, or "gross," although these were all foods he would eat at home. His mother reported that she had approximately 10 foods she knew he would eat regularly: pasta with white cream sauce or butter, pizza from the local pizzeria, bagels lightly toasted with nothing on them, bananas, applesauce, a particular sweet breakfast cereal, cheddar cheese sticks, potato chips of a few different varieties, white bread with butter, and most desserts. His intake generally represented rotations of these foods and little else. On rare occasions he would try another food. **His mother admitted she no longer even tried to present new foods to Jo because he would become anxious, tearful, and irritable and would begin to cry and lose his temper.** The family viewed these behaviors as unusual in the family; Jo's two siblings are more typical eaters.

The reason for presentation at the clinic at this time was due to weight loss at his pediatrics visit and a **subsequent 9 months of follow-up with his doctor to help support weight gain.** Jo's mother felt his weight loss was likely due to his recent growth spurt and taking up soccer, with practice twice a week and games on weekends. She felt that with Jo's intake, it was **very challenging to keep up with his nutritional needs.** She had taken to packing a hot lunch and delivering it to him at school each day, often pulling him from class to eat with him as he took an unusually long time to eat. Jo's mother reported that, if she did not monitor, it was assumed he would try it but not finish it. The doctor had suggested that the family **work with a nutritionist,** and they had 10 visits. The family stopped services because they felt these were not helpful; the nutritionist outlined goals for healthy eating, but Jo would not eat these foods, and Jo's mother felt increasingly **guilty that she was unable to provide sufficiently for her son.**

The family was also **referred to an occupational therapy (OT) specialist,** who determined that Jo had normal eating behaviors but an extremely limited range of foods and a "sensitive palate." They had seen the OT three times at the time of presentation, and she had made a suggestion that they come to the eating disorders clinic for behavioral assistance and to rule out other psychiatric causes of his limited intake.

The intake revealed that **Jo had significant areas of worry around foods "not tasting good" and not wanting to eat something he did not like.** He was **not at all concerned about his body weight or shape;** indeed, he wanted to gain weight and felt uncomfortable at his lower weight and as other boys had started to tease him for being small. He was upset that his mother came to school for lunch, preferring instead to be able to play with his friends, and he became tearful when his mother interrupted and noted that he was not responsible enough to eat his lunch on his own. He reported that he would eat more if his parents gave him foods he liked and stopped insisting he had to eat things that were "gross" or "disgusting." He reported not listening to the dietitian since "she just talked to my mom, and I didn't care what they were talking about," and he felt his doctor's concern around his weight was caused by his mom being "too worried." Jo's mother acknowledged her ongoing worry and noted that they had tried so many things, had read "every book on the subject of feeding children," and that "nothing worked." At times, such as the past 9 months when they were more concerned, **the family would engage in heightened battles around increasing intake, while at other times they would "just relax and try to go with it, because all this worry about food isn't helping anyone."** The family wanted guidance on how to effectively feed Jo, what divisions of responsibility should be around increasing and maintaining intake. They also wanted to increase his weight as they were concerned about him falling off of his growth curve.

Sarah—Disrupted Homeostatic Appetite

Sarah, age 6, presented to the eating disorders clinic for an intake. She had been seen in rheumatology for early onset of juvenile rheumatoid arthritis (JRA), which was diagnosed at age 5. Both parents were physicians and caught symptoms early. Sarah had been undergoing a variety of medical procedures, and the family had recently started using methotrexate to help control symptoms. While this was effective in controlling JRA, Sarah complained of frequent pain, stomach upset, and fatigue. Her team was concerned as she was very small for her age; falling at the **5th percentile for height and no longer on the growth chart for weight.** Initially her treatment team felt her weight was due to her physical discomfort, but in reviewing with the parents, they identified that **Sarah had never had a large appetite,** and often would eat very little in a sitting. When she was younger, they simply thought this was a typical toddler appetite, but as her younger sister met and then exceeded Sarah's growth, the family became concerned. When her much younger sister also met and exceeded Sarah's growth, the family became very concerned. The treatment team also become concerned that Sarah's low weight was impacting her treatment, placing her at increasing risk for other challenges, particularly as she started showing difficulties with Reynaud's syndrome.

When discussing eating behaviors, the parents noted two things: Sarah "eats like a bird"—she might take four or five small bites of a food and then say she was "full" or "done." She was simply **disinterested in food** and had started making comments that she "hated eating" and thought having to eat meals was "stupid." She was also quite limited in the range of food she wanted to eat, and her parents found she was becoming more and more strident in her rejection of foods she did not want to eat. For example, she would only eat one piece of pizza but without any sauce and only with a specific cheese on it. During this discussion she turned to her parents and said, "If they try to give it to you with sauce, you tell them 'ABSOLUTELY NOT.'" Parents had **worked with OT,** both as part of her JRA and to address eating via exposure therapy. During these sessions, **Sarah would be sometimes willing to try something, but this did not carry over to trying things at home,** despite the family's efforts. Her parents recruited help at school to have someone eat lunch with Sarah, brought specific foods and snacks that they felt she liked the best, and attempted to make eating "fun and entertaining" for her. The family reported that **Sarah's preferences limited what each person in the family could eat,** as her parents did not want to cook and serve multiple meals. The parents worried about Sarah's **faltering weight and the impact on her health, but also the impact on her siblings,** who had also started raising objections to eating certain foods. They were concerned that **they struggled to get her to increase her intake at all,** even by as little as one or two bites more, as she simply would sit and stare at the food and refuse to take another bite. They tried to wait it out, as suggested by the OT specialist. They had tried to provide rewards, but these often fell flat after the first few times. They tried to provide a wide variety of food and help Sarah sample new foods. Sarah was not upset about eating; she ate a variety of different foods but simply seemed to **not have any appetite or desire to eat.**

Josie—Choking and Vomiting Phobia

Josie, a 13-year-old female, presented to her pediatrician's office with rapid weight loss and significantly attenuated eating. Her mother requested the evaluation, stating that Josie had **suddenly started refusing to eat solid foods.** After meeting with their pediatrician, they were referred to an eating disorders evaluation for what the pediatrician felt was likely AN. In meeting with the family and gathering history on Josie's eating, the family indicated the following.

She had **no previous eating difficulties** and was a normally developing young woman. She had started her menses 4 months prior, indicating appropriate growth and development and had **not expressed any body image concerns currently or in the past.** She denied concerns about her physical development or puberty. The family reported that 5 months prior, the family had been on vacation in Israel and she had **choked on an apple.** Her brother, thinking quickly, performed the Heimlich maneuver and dislodged the apple slice. She also vomited at that time. She experienced a sore rib and a "scratchy throat" but no other ill effects. Her parents noted that she refused to eat apples but felt that was a rather appropriate reaction to this trauma.

When the family returned home, they noticed that Josie was more particular about eating, often serving herself **smaller portions and taking a long time chewing and eating her food.** They also noticed that she would **ask for softer foods,** such as soups or mashed potatoes. The family was happy to comply with these requests, as Josie had never had any previous eating concerns. Over the next 2 weeks they noticed that she started **to cut out more and more solid foods,** drinking soup broth but leaving the more nourishing aspects of the soup in the bowl. When the family went to a family dinner, Josie became tearful when her grandmother served a beef brisket and carrots. Josie refused to eat. Her parents encouraged her to mash up the carrots, but even this appeared to be too much for her, and she became tearful. The next day, Josie made herself a smoothie from milk and a banana. For dinner she did the same. From that point forward this seemed to be her more typical daily routine. She told her parents she was eating lunch at school, but when asked, she could not say what she had had besides milk. Four months later, she had **lost more than 20 pounds and met criteria for bradycardia.** Following her meeting with eating disorder outpatient clinic staff, Josie was hospitalized for her bradycardia at an eating disorders clinic.

In the hospital, the eating disorders team evaluated her intake and observed the following: Josie was **afraid of choking on foods much larger than one-eighth of an inch.** However, since she could not always tell what was in a food, she would reject all foods that might have pieces larger than this. Additionally, she was concerned about eating foods that had peels, apart from a banana, where the peel was easily and totally removed, because as she was **concerned that these might stick in her throat.** She was **willing to eat high-calorie-density foods,** including whole-fat dairy, butter, full-fat yogurt, and mashed potatoes, but would become fearful before each meal and would ask repeatedly about what was in her food. She was receptive to relaxation introduced prior to meals, and this helped her increase her intake sufficiently to halt weight loss and improve stability. She was **receptive to high-calorie supplementation.** She was able to practice increasingly larger portion sizes and was discharged from the hospital in 7 days with the expectation that she would return to eating at home. A swallow study revealed no physiological impediments to eating.

The family struggled to increase her intake at home, finding that she could maintain eating the foods that were introduced in the hospital but struggled to return to her typical eating. She was maintaining, even gaining, but on largely a liquid diet. The family requested behavioral treatment to help increase her weight.

Evidence-Based Outpatient Treatments for Avoidant/Restrictive Food Intake Disorder

There are no evidence-based treatments for ARFID. The following approaches are considered experimental approaches (Level 4).

- Family-based treatment
- Cognitive-behavioral therapy
- Exposure prevention therapy
- Behavioral therapy

Treatment

There are no evidenced-based practice parameters for ARFID. To date, treatment methods have been outlined in case series or small treatment trials. Data are being collected from several different randomized controlled trials of ARFID across the age range. Results from these studies will likely be available by 2022. Experimental treatments have generally focused on three core areas: sensory-based food exposures, anxiety management techniques, and significant support in increasing intake at each meal (e.g., parent-based support, residential/partial-hospital/intensive-outpatient support). Patients with ARFID have been seen in eating disorder clinics and treatment facilities, and many are now offering specific services for those presenting with ARFID, although without specific guidelines to drive treatment. All treatment levels may utilize psychology, psychiatry, and occupational and physical therapy to enhance eating behaviors

Outpatient programs have often seen children who are presenting with ARFID, including eating, pain, and consultation-liaison services. Depending on the unique view of the clinic, most outpatient programs bring a mix of anxiety and pain management, and exposure therapies to support enhanced eating. Treatments typically used include adapted versions of family-based treatment (FBT) and cognitive-behavioral therapy (CBT).

Self-help books targeting parents and eating behaviors are one of the most popular arenas to provide information on ARFID. These range from books on reinforcing the importance of a wide range of foods from toddlerhood to adulthood, to those specifically covering "extreme picky eating," to those addressing choking and vomiting phobias. Books have been written by parents, sociologists, speech pathologists/occupational therapists, psychologists, and developmental behaviorists.

Hospitalization has been utilized in ARFID when there is significant malnourishment and when medical issues require ongoing evaluation and monitoring for patient safety (e.g., to avoid refeeding syndrome, to address severe weight loss). Patients may be seen in main hospital clinics, often presenting to consultation/liaison or psychosomatic service divisions, as well as in more traditional eating disorder programs. To assist with weight gain, some hospitals place nasogastric and gastrostomy tubes to support ongoing renourishment efforts. It should be noted that withdrawal of feeding tubes should be done slowly and with specific behavioral markers for success (Dovey et al. 2017).

Residential treatment facilities, partial hospitalization programs (PHPs), and intensive outpatient programs (IOPs) have long had ARFID patients whose symptoms meet criteria for restricted eating as well as low weight, and there has been a history of accepting these patients and encouraging weight restoration through increasing intake. Many programs utilize anxiety management and exposure therapies to support enhanced eating.

Although there are no evidence-based treatments for ARFID, we discuss two likely candidate treatments, FBT and CBT, in more detail, and they are approaches that are currently being studied and used clinically.

Family-Based Treatment for Avoidant/ Restrictive Food Intake Disorder

As noted, many of the patients with ARFID are children and adolescents. Thus, it is not surprising that treatment might include parents when these younger patients do not require inpatient care. Although there is not yet substantive evidence supporting a family-based approach, there is a rationale for considering this type of treatment might be effective. The theoretical understanding or overall philosophy of this approach is that the child is embedded in the family and that the parents' involvement in therapy is vitally important for ultimate success in treatment. In ARFID, the child is often seen as regressed or immature. Therefore, parents should be involved in their offspring's treatment, while showing respect and regard for their child's point of view and experience.

FBT for ARFID pays close attention to developmental and sensory issues and aims to guide the parents eventually to assist their child with age-appropriate tasks. During this process, fundamental work on other family conflicts or disagreements has to be deferred until the eating disorder behaviors are out of the way. Normal development is seen as having been arrested and severely impacted by the presence of the eating disorder. The parents are temporarily put in charge to help reduce the hold ARFID has over the child's and the family's life. Once successful in this task, the parents will help the child gain more age-appropriate control and assist them in the usual negotiation of predictable childhood adolescent development tasks, as applicable.

FBT for ARFID differs from other treatments of patients with eating disorders in several key ways. First, as pointed out, the child is not viewed as being in control of his or her behavior; instead, ARFID controls it. Thus, in this way only, the child is seen as functioning not at an age-appropriate level but instead as a much younger child who is in need of a great deal of help from the parents. Second, the treatment aims to correct this position by not only improving parental control over the child's eating but, at the same time, helping the child explore new textures, flavors, smells, colors, and types of food. In the FBT view, parental control and self-efficacy have often been lost because parents might feel that they are to blame for their child's ARFID or the symptoms have frightened them to the extent that they are too afraid to act decisively. Third, the FBT approach strongly advocates that the therapist should primarily focus his or her attention on the tasks of weight restoration, reduced anxiety around eating, and increasing variety of food consumed, particularly in the early parts of treatment. This approach, therefore, tends to "stay with the eating disorder" for longer—that is, the therapist remains alert so as not to become distracted from the central therapeutic task, which is to keep the parents focused on expanding their child's eating so as to free them from the control of the eating disorder.

Phase 1: Charging the Parents With the Task of Renourishment and Coaching Them During This Task (Sessions 1–10)

In phase 1 (Table 5–1), the main goal of the treatment is to align both parents on the serious and urgent duty of breaking the behavioral patterns associated with ARFID. To achieve this, the therapist uses therapeutic strategies such as psychoeducation, externalization of ARFID symptoms, and a family meal session to observe and coach feeding strategies. Throughout the meetings, the role of the parental unit in facilitating the change in their child's ARFID symptoms is emphasized, while the parents and the siblings are encouraged to support the child as he or she develops anxiety reduction skills around eating.

Phase 2: Helping the Child to Eat More Independently (Sessions 11–15)

The mood displayed by the therapist in phase 2 is different from the somber and sad tone characteristic of most of phase 1. By the time the family moves into phase 2, the patient and the family would have demonstrated progress in terms of weight regain or management of specific nutritional deficiencies. This advance should be reflected in the therapist's mood when he or she embarks on this next step in treatment. In addition, unlike the more structured nature of treatment interventions concerning refeeding the child up to this point, guidelines for the

TABLE 5–1. Outline of family-based treatment for avoidant/restrictive food intake disorder (ARFID)

Phase (meetings)	Therapeutic focus
Phase 1, sessions 1–10	*Main goal:* Charging and coaching the parents with the task of renourishment
	• Keep the family focused on the eating disorder
	• Help the parents take responsibility for their child's eating
	• Mobilize siblings to support the patient
	• Use psychoeducation and externalization of ARFID symptoms to reduce criticism
	• Include a family meal session to observe and coach feeding strategies
Phase 2, sessions 11–15	*Main goal:* Helping the child eat on more independently
	• Maintain parental management of ARFID symptoms until the patient shows evidence of greater mastery in eating novel foods in sufficient amounts
	• Expand exposures to facilitate greater flexibility in age-appropriate eating
	• Explore relationship between developmental issues and ARFID
Phase 3, sessions 15–20	*Main goal:* Identifying potential future challenges and improving resilience
	• Establish a child-parent relationship that is substantial beyond communication around ARFID
	• Review developmental issues and model problem solving
	• Create a plan for relapse prevention and terminate treatment.

therapist's style/technique from here onward are less circumscribed. From a developmental perspective, the eating disorder can be seen as having "interfered" with the patient's normal development. Therefore, the therapist's task now is to help get the patient "back into" normal trajectories while helping the family identify and reduce the maintaining factors that reinforce ARFID symptoms. It should be noted that the parents also need to develop a normal trajectory mindset—that is, they need to adopt the notion of their child growing up and assuming greater autonomy. The specifics of this process are highly individualistic, and there is seldom a prescribed way to proceed. Instead, we provide broad guidelines about therapeutic procedures the therapist should begin to introduce toward the latter part of this treatment phase.

Phase 3: Identifying Potential Future Challenges and Improving Resilience (Sessions 16–20)

Phase 3 is initiated when the patient achieves a stable weight, the extent of anxiety and avoidance around eating new foods has abated, and control over eating has been continuously returned to the child in a way that is suitable with age and comorbidities. The central theme in this phase is the establishment of a healthy relationship between child and parents in which the illness does not constitute the basis of interaction. This entails, among other things, working toward increased autonomy and mastery for the child, setting and maintaining appropriate intergenerational family boundaries, and recognizing the need for the parents to reorganize their lives as a family with the declined impact of ARFID. Attention to parental professional and leisure interests is a legitimate focus of this phase.

Cognitive-Behavioral Treatment for Avoidant/Restrictive Food Intake Disorder

There is to date no published manual or protocol specific for the treatment of ARFID using CBT. However, the main authors of the approach have argued that the approach is transdiagnostic—that is, applicable to all eating disorder diagnoses (Fairburn et al. 2002, 2008). Some data about the effectiveness of CBT across diagnoses—AN, BN, binge-eating disorder (BED), and eating disorders that do not meet full criteria for a specific diagnosis—are available (Fairburn et al. 2009), but no data are specifically available for ARFID.

There are reasons to consider that CBT might be effective for ARFID because dietary restriction and anxiety about eating are characteristics shared with more traditional eating disorders and ARFID (Bryant-Waugh and Kreipe 2012). In addition, both more typical eating disorders and ARFID are accompanied by a range of cognitive distortions (Fairburn and Bohn 2005). On the other hand, because patients with ARFID do not have shape and weight concerns and do not engage in behaviors to address worries about these factors, many of the typical interventions used in CBT likely would not apply. At the same time, data suggest that behavioral interventions in CBT lead to changes (Fairburn et al. 1996)—that is, developing and maintaining a normal eating pattern (three meals and two or three snacks), monitoring dietary behaviors through keeping food records, and taking up eating challenging or avoided foods. In addition to these observations, it is important to note that research on CBT for eating disorders has mostly focused on adults, whereas many if not most of the patients with ARFID are children and adolescents.

CBT approaches have been used for other child and adolescent mental health problems, such as depression, anxiety, and obsessive-compulsive disorder, and been shown to be effective (Barrett 1998; Brent et al. 1997; Cooper and Stewart 2008; Kolko et al. 2000; Walkup et al. 2008; Weisz et al. 2009). However, with younger patients, parents are usually highly involved in the process, supporting the structure of behavioral and emotional challenges and supporting their children's treatment directly (Le Grange et al. 2015; Lock 2005).

When we consider these observations as a whole, a CBT approach for ARFID will likely be parent led or guided, especially for younger patients, and focus on behavior changes specific to the type of ARFID rather than addressing cognitive change. In addition, developmental considerations in terms of cognitive, emotional, and social maturity and needs would be a component in adapting CBT for ARFID (CBT-ARFID) (Lock 2005). Thus, phase 1 of CBT-ARFID would likely involve enlisting the parents' support and involvement in trying to change the maintaining behaviors of ARFID (undereating, fearful eating, extreme picky eating) in their child. CBT would typically employ psychoeducation about the likely consequences—medical, emotional, and social—of these maintaining behaviors. Next, parents would be asked to either directly monitor (if it is a child who is too young or one who is unwilling) or begin monitoring eating and keeping a record of the child's eating with the aim of promoting a more normal eating pattern. The specific focus in early sessions would be reviewing these food records with the child and parent to identify problematic areas such as undereating, overeating, limited range of foods eaten, and mood state (particularly anxiety) when preparing to eat or eating. Once clear behavioral targets (i.e., maintaining behaviors) are identified, specific strategies would be discussed with the parent and child to begin to challenge specific maintaining behaviors. The second stage of ARFID would focus on challenging these behaviors with the goal of weight gain (if the patient is underweight), expanding food range (if the patient is a picky eater), or overcoming anxiety about eating (if the patient is overcoming a traumatic swallowing, allergic, or related problem). In addition, in this stage, CBT-ARFID would focus on continuing to expand the target behaviors (eating more, eating a greater variety, eating without fear or anxiety) and generalizing eating in typical child and adolescent environments where eating takes place (e.g., school, friend's homes, parties). The final stage of CBT-ARFID would focus on relapse prevention—that is, identifying potential stresses that could lead to relapse to help the parents develop a plan to intervene should such stressors arise.

It is worth noting that in cases in which individuals with ARFID first present in adolescence or adulthood or when treatment is with this age group, a CBT approach would likely be very different, with parents taking a much more supportive role rather than actively promoting behavioral change. In addition, there would likely be an opportunity to use more cognitive aspects of CBT than would be used with younger patients to address cognitive distortions and to challenge beliefs. While these would not focus on shape and weight issues, as would be the case when CBT is used with AN, BN, and BED, issues related to unrealistic fears and anxieties about eating, particular foods, classes of foods, and eating beyond fullness might well be subject to cognitive therapy.

Treatments Illustrated

As noted, there are no evidence-based treatments for ARFID. We choose to illustrate here FBT approaches for the three main presentations of ARFID in children because this approach is currently being researched and a basic manual is available that outlines the approach (Fitzpatrick et al. 2015).

Family-Based Treatment for Low Appetite

Alice is a 6-year-old girl whose parents have brought her to treatment for ARFID because she is no longer on a reasonable growth curve. Her pediatrician is concerned and has discussed the possibility of tube feeding if she does not increase her weight. Alice was born prematurely and required tube feeding as an infant. Subsequently, she has continued throughout her short life to have a low appetite and has been in lowest growth percentiles for height and weight throughout her childhood. In contrast, her younger sister, who is 5 years old, is taller and weighs more. Parents say that Alice is a wonderful child but that she just has no interest in eating. She would rather play or read than eat. She is easily distracted from eating and will often talk or play rather than eat at the table. Alice eats a full range of foods and does not actively avoid foods with fats or carbohydrates. Parents have been reluctant to push hard for Alice to eat because their own parents forced them to "clean their plates," and they did not think this was helpful to them.

FBT for ARFID (FBT-ARFID) begins with a first session in which the current medical, social, and emotional issues that accompany ARFID are identified and discussed by the entire family. The purpose of this session is to get the parents on the same page and to agree to take action to change the status quo of undereating. To accomplish this goal, the therapist engages the entire family in a discussion of how Alice's undereating is affecting her and the family. The parents report that because of Alice's eating patterns the family spends many hours at the dinner table rather than doing other things, argues about eating and eating enough, and worries constantly about the health impacts of undereating on Alice. Using this information, the therapist tries to incite the parents to action. The therapist acknowledges that the family has "accommodated" or adjusted their lives to adapt to Alice's undereating and that it may be difficult to see a way forward, but it is essential for Alice's future health and well-being that things change. The therapist is careful not to blame the parents for their past decisions related to Alice's eating and to promote the understanding that Alice is also not to blame for having a low appetite. Instead, the therapist externalizes ARFID and asks the family to fight it together. The session concludes with the therapist summarizing the session, then asking the family to bring a meal for the next session that they think will help Alice gain weight.

The family arrives on time for the second session, and the session begins as the family lays out the meal. The meal they have brought consists of sandwiches, chips, fruit juice, and cookies. Everyone begins eating, but the therapist notes that Alice is slower to start and eats very slowly compared with everyone else. In part, this is because she is talking to her sister or her parents. The therapist asks the parents how they decided on this meal, and they reported it was a typical lunch for them. When asked how much Alice typically ate of this meal, the parents indicate about half or a little less. The therapist asks if they think she needs to eat more than that, and they readily say that they think so. At this point, the therapist asks the parents to discuss how they would like to help Alice eat more. At first the parents are a bit confused, but with a little coaching from the therapist, they decide that she should finish her sandwich and eat some of the cookie. Knowing what they want her to eat is a key first step. The therapist next asks the parents to encourage Alice to eat what they agreed needed to be eaten. Alice's mother asks Alice to try to eat more while her father sits quietly. Alice does not eat more. The therapist suggests that if both parents tell, not ask, Alice to eat, she might eat. The difference between "asking" and "telling" is highlighted by the therapist, because it is important for Alice to know that there is no choice in the matter. Alice begins to eat a little of the sandwich, and the therapist compliments her on listening to her parents, who are trying to help her be stronger and grow. The parents also reinforce Alice by saying they are happy she is eating. The remainder of the session is spent helping the parents try different approaches to encouraging Alice to eat. By the conclusion of the session, Alice has eaten most of her sandwich and has taken a bite of a cookie. The therapist praises the family and encourages them to continue to do the things they have learned in session at home until they meet the following week.

During the following weeks, Alice and her family come to therapy weekly. At the beginning of every session, Alice is weighed and her weight is plotted on a graph so that she and the family can see the progress she is making. At first, Alice gains weight slowly, but as the family finds ways to help her eat more, she begins to have a steady upward curve in her weight. One of the main challenges the family face is the amount of time it takes for Alice to eat. It sometimes takes close to 2 hours for dinner to be consumed. This process is exhausting for the parents and also very hard on Alice. A plan is devised to use a timer for each meal and to reward completing the meal on time with additional play time, screen time, or social time with the parents. This works well overall, though the parents' reluctance to push Alice because of their own family histories interferes at times with the rate of change. Still in about 3 months, the pediatrician is pleased with the progress and stops seeing Alice regularly. Alice has surpassed her previous growth curve. She still needs encouragement to eat enough—her appetite, though improved, is not a reliable guide for her eating, so her parents are expected to continue to need to help her eat enough over the next several years.

Family-Based Treatment for Selective Eating

Most children who present with ARFID associated with severe selective or "picky" eating are also underweight, though not dramatically so, and often appear poorly nourished because the range of foods they eat do not provide them with required nutrients for health. Michael, in the following case, is such a boy.

Michael is 10 years old, bright, and precocious intellectually. He is the second oldest of three siblings in an intact family. Michael's parents work out of their home and also homeschool their children. Michael is a good student, but he has low energy much of the time and is sometimes moody and irritable. According to his mother, Michael has been a picky eater since he began eating solid food, preferring bland, starchy foods and avoiding fruits and vegetables and most meats. Although Michael is not really stunted in his growth, he is small and thin. His appearance contrasts markedly with his brother, who is 2 years older than him and is tall, robust, and athletic looking.

As in FBT for low-weight ARFID, the beginning of therapy aims to incite the parents to make decisive changes related to eating behaviors. To do this, the developmental, social, and emotional impact of poor nutrition are emphasized in the first session. The therapist tries to instill a sense of urgency while acknowledging that Michael has been a long-time picky eater. To help the family identify and characterize Michael's current eating, the therapist introduces asks the family to devise a list of foods that Michael eats "always" and "sometimes" and those he "never" eats but that would be helpful to the family if he did. Michael helps with generating these lists. This list serves as a kind of therapeutic scaffold, with the aim of moving more foods into the "sometimes" and "always" list and reducing the "never" list. The session ends by asking the parents to bring a meal to the next session that includes items from each of the categories on the list. As is the case with FBT for all disorders, parents are specifically not blamed for having done anything to cause ARFID, and the patient is similarly not blamed for being a selective eater. Instead, ARFID is externalized as an illness, thereby allowing the family to confront the problematic eating behavior without feelings of guilt.

Michael's parents bring a peanut butter and jelly sandwich, chips, and water for Michael to eat. In addition to peanut butter sandwiches, they bring milk, carrots, and chocolate cookies for his younger sister and older brother. Milk and carrots are on Michael's "never" list, and the cookies are on his "sometimes" list. As expected, Michael eats his sandwich with little difficulty but struggles to try the carrots and refuses the milk entirely. He eats a bit of the cookie after his brother tells him how good it is. The therapist asks Michael's parents why they have brought carrots and milk. They explain that they feel Michael needs to drink milk—he is not allergic to it, they emphasize—to help him grow. Carrots they say are a vegetable that is common at lots of sports events and practices, so it would be good to be able to eat them. The therapist asks the parents to prioritize which food they would like to focus on. They decide they would like for Michael to try to drink some milk. Michael protests strongly that he hates milk and always has, but they remind him that he often has had milk in things—like cereal and milkshakes. Trying to reason with Michael does not work, however. The therapist suggests they decide what they would be satisfied with today. They would be happy with a single sip. Michael agrees and takes one. He spits out most of the milk but then tries again as his parents encouraged him. The therapist praises him and the parents for sticking with this and asks them to begin to try some of the things on the "sometimes" list during the week between sessions.

During the first phase of FBT-ARFID for selective eating, the goal is to gradually increase the food range. It is important not to overwhelm the patient and family with really challenging foods at the beginning, and it is good to build on success. For example, Michael tries the milk, but an entire glass of milk is really overwhelming for him. Instead, if the milk were to be flavored with chocolate, he would drink more of it. Other foods with milk in them are gradually added to Michael's repertoire. Unlike FBT for AN, where early in treatment the patient is not usually able to be constructive, in FBT-ARFID, the patient can often be very helpful by suggesting what foods he or she would like to try next and what kinds of incentives would be most helpful. Within a few weeks, the family notices Michael was less moody and irritable and attributes this to his eating more and more nutritious foods. This is a real possibility, and the therapist encourages this perspective.

FBT for AN or BN usually is for adolescents, but FBT-ARFID often involves much younger children who are not yet embarking on adolescence. The third of phase of FBT-ARFID therefore does not usually focus on adolescent issues as it would for AN or BN. Instead, the third phase of FBT-ARFID is focused mostly on how the family can continue to make progress after treatment ends and relapse prevention.

This was the case with Michael, who is a very young 10-year-old physically and emotionally. During the third phase, the therapist helps the family summarize the progress they have made—how many foods have been moved from the "never" to the "sometimes" and the "sometimes" to the "always" list, Michael's height and weight increase, and his mood improves. They decide on what other foods they want to work on in the future and agree to avoid "slipping back."

Family-Based Therapy for Fear of Swallowing After Trauma

FBT for ARFID of acute onset after trauma most resembles FBT for AN because, unlike ARFID associated with low appetite or highly selective eating, this presentation is a marked departure from previous behaviors, as in AN. Most children with AN were eating normally before developing AN, and parents and other family members can clearly remember this and articulate the changes that came about as AN developed. Similarly, for ARFID that develops acutely after some form of injury or trauma, parents and family members can readily distinguish the eating behaviors before the trauma and after. In some ways, this makes working with ARFID related to a trauma easier, because the family has not had many years of accommodating to either low appetite or picky eating. The health impacts are also often more clearly apparent with the acute-onset posttraumatic version of ARFID because weight loss is sometimes rapid.

Lucy is an 11-year-girl who choked on a piece of pizza at a friend's party several months ago and who subsequently refused to eat solid foods of any type for fear of choking again. She has reduced her intake further to only clear liquids, like broths, out of fear that thicker soups or small vegetables might cause her to choke. Even with these clear broths, though, Lucy sometimes chokes and spits them out because, as she says, "they stick in my throat." Lucy has lost almost 20 pounds over the past several months and is weak and lethargic. She is too tired to go to school and has withdrawn from her friends except through social media.

When the family arrives for the first session of FBT-ARFID for this extreme fear of swallowing, they are all visibly anxious about coming. Lucy's mother has called several times to make sure that Lucy's brother should attend because Lucy does not like for him to hear about her problems. The therapist assures her that Lucy's brother would be important to include, given that he is a part of the family, and that his perspective and needs also need to be addressed. Lucy's father is concerned about missing work because he has already been away from work because of Lucy's medical appointment, and he feels his wife is the one who is "in charge" of eating in their house. The therapist insists that the success of Lucy's treatment depends on both parents being present and says that it would not be possible to conduct FBT without him. He reluctantly agrees to attend.

The therapist meets with Lucy before the first session and weighs her. Lucy is very thin and pale with dark hair. She is friendly and soft spoken. The therapist explains that this therapy is about helping her overcome her fear of eating and to get her back to where she was before the choking incident. Lucy is tearful and says that she is not sure that anything can help. After weighing Lucy, the therapist calls the family into the office and asks each member of the family to briefly introduce himself or herself. After these introductions, the therapist asks the family as a whole to describe what has happened to the family since Lucy choked on the pizza several months before. Lucy's father begins by saying that he has observed Lucy avoid eating solid foods, not eat thick liquids, and be anxious about swallowing even clear broth. The problem is getting worse, not better. Lucy's mother agrees with these observations and adds that Lucy is not sleeping well and seems very depressed. Mark, Lucy's brother, says the whole family is sad now because they are worried about Lucy all the time. He says he also cannot sleep sometimes because he is afraid Lucy could die if she does not eat more. The therapist uses this information to illustrate how serious ARFID is—that it has changed Lucy and changed the way the family communicates, and that it would be a threat to Lucy's life if it were to continue. Lucy begins to cry and says that she is sorry. The therapist is quick to point out that no one blames Lucy and that she needs help. Lucky for her, her family loves her and is willing to help. It will likely not be easy, but the therapist is hopeful that Lucy can recover. The therapist next challenges the parents to bring a meal to the next session that is not all liquid but that includes some of the things Lucy is comfortable swallowing.

Unlike FBT for AN, fear of choking is based on a real traumatic event. It is important to respect this when trying to help a patient overcome this fear and not expect the fear to abate immediately. It is also not usually helpful to "flood" the person by insisting they eat only solid foods. A more gradual desensitization exposure program is usually effective. The challenge families face is that they get stopped in their tracks by the fear their child expresses and are reluctant to challenge it because they are afraid they will hurt or damage their child emotionally or physically. This was the case for Lucy's family to a significant extent.

Lucy's mother is protective of Lucy and fears that "forcing" her will make matters worse. While Lucy's father feels Lucy needs to try to eat more normally, he feels he cannot interfere with his wife's hesitancy because she is the one at home taking care of Lucy. These differences become apparent in the meal session. The parents bring clear broth, a vegetable and fruit "smoothie," and some chocolate pudding for Lucy. Lucy finishes the clear broth without too much difficulty but is unwilling to try even a sip of the smoothie. She is tearful and wailing at times. The therapist asks the parents to work together to assure Lucy and say they believe that she can swallow a small sip of the smoothie and that they need her to try. Sitting on either side of her, the parents together hold the smoothie cup with a straw in it for Lucy, and finally she takes a little bit into her mouth. She promptly spits this out, however. The therapist praises Lucy for trying and encourages the parents to try again. Lucy ultimately swallows a bit of the smoothie, and although she does not choke, she remains very upset. The therapist asks Lucy's brother if he might do something to help Lucy feel better. At first, he is flummoxed, but then he pulls out his phone and plays a funny video he has seen earlier in the day. Lucy cannot help but smile at it.

The first step is the hardest in overcoming fear of choking. Thus, during the following week, as the parents gradually increase the amounts of thick liquids Lucy needs to consume, Lucy's anxiety and fear diminish. Over the course of the first phase of FBT, Lucy progresses from clear broths to smoothies and thick soups, to mashed vegetables, and then carefully chopped meats. Lucy's weight steadily increases, and her mood improves. She once again is involved with friends, and by the end of treatment she is eating normally.

Common Outcomes and Complications

- Both short- and long-term outcomes are unknown.

- It would be expected that earlier treatment can and should result in a reduction of symptoms, but it is unclear the extent to which dietary gains are maintained and this disorder remits.

- Left untreated or poorly treated, those with ARFID will continue to struggle throughout adulthood.

- Evaluations of adult patients with ARFID indicate that many adults simply become more effective at finding ways to meet their nutritional needs or find adaptations that work with their lifestyles.

Resources and Further Reading

Training Resources

CBT: Oxford Cognitive Therapy Centre: https://www.octc.co.uk/training
FBT: Training Institute for Child and Adolescent Eating Disorders: train2treat4ed.com

Further Reading

Brewerton TD, D'Agostino M: Adjunctive use of olanzapine in the treatment of avoidant restrictive food intake disorder in children and adolescents in an eating disorders program. J Child Adolesc Psychopharmacol 27(10):920–922, 2017

Cardona Cano S, Hoek HW, Bryant-Waugh R: Picky eating: the current state of research. Curr Opin Psychiatry 28(6):448–454, 2015

Eddy KT, Thomas JJ, Hastings E, et al: Prevalence of DSM-5 avoidant/restrictive food intake disorder in a pediatric gastroenterology healthcare network. Int J Eat Disord 48(5):464–470, 2015

Fairburn CG: Cognitive Behavior Therapy and Eating Disorders. New York, Guilford, 2008

Lock J, LeGrange D: Treatment Manual for Anorexia Nervosa: A Family-Based Approach, 2nd Edition. New York, Guilford, 2013

Norris ML, Spettigue W, Hammond NG, et al: Building evidence for the use of descriptive subtypes in youth with avoidant restrictive food intake disorder. Int J Eat Disord 51(2)170–173, 2018

Thomas, J, Lawson, EA, Micali M, et al: Avoidant/restrictive food intake disorder: a three-dimensional model of neurobiology with implications for etiology and treatment. Curr Psychiatry Rep 19(8):54, 2017

Zickgraf HF, Franklin ME, Rozin P: Adult picky eaters with symptoms of avoidant/restrictive food intake disorder: comparable distress and comorbidity but different eating behaviors compared to those with disordered eating symptoms. J Eat Disord 4:26, 2016

References

American Psychiatric Association: Diagnostic and Statistical Manual of Mental Disorders, 4th Edition, Text Revision. Washington, DC, American Psychiatric Association, 2000

American Psychiatric Association: Diagnostic and Statistical Manual of Mental Disorders, 5th Edition. Arlington, VA, American Psychiatric Association, 2013

Barrett PM: Evaluation of cognitive-behavioral group treatments for childhood anxiety disorders. J Clin Child Psychol 27(4):459–468, 1998 9866083

Brent DA, Holder D, Kolko D, et al: A clinical psychotherapy trial for adolescent depression comparing cognitive, family, and supportive therapy. Arch Gen Psychiatry 54(9):877–885, 1997 9294380

Bryant-Waugh R, Kreipe R: Avoidant/Restrictive food intake disorder in DSM-5. Psychiatr Ann 42(11):402–405, 2012

Bryant-Waugh R, Markham L, Kreipe RE, et al: Feeding and eating disorders in childhood. Int J Eat Disord 43(2):98–111, 2010 20063374

Bryant-Waugh R, Nicholls D (eds): Diagnosis and Classification of Disordered Eating in Childhood. New York, Guilford, 2011

Cardona Cano S, Hoek HW, Bryant-Waugh R: Picky eating: the current state of research. Curr Opin Psychiatry 28(6):448–454, 2015 26382157

Cooper Z, Stewart A: CBT-E and the younger patient, in Cognitive Behavioral Therapy and Eating Disorders. Edited by Fairburn CG. New York, Guilford, 2008, pp 221–230

Dovey T, Wilken M, Martin CI, et al: Definitions and clinical guidance on the enteral dependence component of the avoidant/restrictive food intake disorder diagnostic criteria in children. JPEN J Perenter Enteral Nutr July 1, 2017 (Epub ahead of print) 28727947

Eddy KT, Thomas JJ, Hastings E, et al: Prevalence of DSM-5 avoidant/restrictive food intake disorder in a pediatric gastroenterology healthcare network. Int J Eat Disord 48(5):464–470, 2015 25142784

Fairburn CG, Bohn K: Eating disorder NOS (EDNOS): an example of the troublesome "not otherwise specified" (NOS) category in DSM-IV. Behav Res Ther 43(6):691–701, 2005 15890163

Fairburn CG, Marcus MD, Wilson GT: Cognitive-behavioral therapy for binge eating and bulimia nervosa: a comprehensive treatment manual, in Binge Eating: Nature, Assessment, and Treatment. Edited by Fairburn CG, Wilson GT. New York, Guilford, 1996, pp 361–404

Fairburn CG, Cooper Z, Shafran R: Cognitive behavioral therapy for eating disorders: a "transdiagnostic" theory and treatment. Behav Res Ther 41(5):509–528, 2002

Fairburn CG, Cooper Z, Shafran R: Enhanced cognitive behavioral therapy for eating disorders ("CBT-E"): an overview, in Cognitive Behavioral Therapy and Eating Disorders. Edited by Fairburn CG. New York, Guilford, 2008, pp 23–34

Fairburn CG, Cooper Z, Doll HA, et al: Transdiagnostic cognitive-behavioral therapy for patients with eating disorders: a two-site trial with 60-week follow-up. Am J Psychiatry 166(3):311–319, 2009 19074978

Fisher MM, Rosen DS, Ornstein RM, et al: Characteristics of avoidant/restrictive food intake disorder in children and adolescents: a "new disorder" in DSM-5. J Adolesc Health 55(1):49–52, 2014 24506978

Fitzpatrick K, Forsberg S, et al: Family based treatment for avoidant restrictive food intake disorder: families facing neophobias, in Family Therapy for Adolescent Eating and Weight Disorders: New Applications. Edited by Loeb K, Le Grange D, Lock J. New York, Routledge, 2015, pp 256–276

Kolko DJ, Brent DA, Baugher M, et al: Cognitive and family therapies for adolescent depression: treatment specificity, mediation, and moderation. J Consult Clin Psychol 68(4):603–614, 2000 10965636

Le Grange D, Lock J, Agras WS, et al: Randomized clinical trial of family based treatment and cognitive-behavioral therapy for adolescent bulimia nervosa. J Am Acad Child Adolesc Psychiatry 54(11):886–894, 2015 26506579

Lock J: Adjusting cognitive behavior therapy for adolescents with bulimia nervosa: results of case series. Am J Psychother 59(3):267–281, 2005 16370133

Nicely TA, Lane-Loney S, Masciulli E, et al: Prevalence and characteristics of avoidant/restrictive food intake disorder in a cohort of young patients in day treatment for eating disorders. J Eat Disord 2(1):21, 2014 25165558

Pinhas L, Nicholls D, Crosby RD, et al: Classification of childhood onset eating disorders: a latent class analysis. Int J Eat Disord 50(6):657–664, 2017 28106914

Thomas J, Lawson E, Micali N, et al: Avoidant/restrictive food intake disorder: a three-dimensional model of neurobiology with implications for etiology and treatment. Curr Psychiatry Rep 19(8):54, 2017

Turner H, Bryant-Waugh R: Eating disorder not otherwise specified (EDNOS) profiles of clients presenting at a community eating disorder service. Eur Eat Disord Rev 12(1):18–26, 2004

Walkup JT, Albano AM, Piacentini J, et al: Cognitive behavioral therapy, sertraline, or a combination in childhood anxiety. N Engl J Med 359(26):2753–2766, 2008 18974308

Weisz JR, Southam-Gerow MA, Gordis EB, et al: Cognitive-behavioral therapy versus usual clinical care for youth depression: an initial test of transportability to community clinics and clinicians. J Consult Clin Psychol 77(3):383–396, 2009 19485581

Chapter 6

Atypical Eating Disorders

Lilya Osipov, Ph.D.

Introduction

This chapter addresses several factors that may impact the detection, assessment, and treatment of eating disorders. The chapter provides an overview of atypical eating disorder presentations that are encountered in clinical practice and their treatments. Frequently, atypical eating disorder presentations go unnoticed because providers do not think to ask about these behaviors or are quick to attribute symptoms to other medical or psychological conditions. The goal of this chapter is to enhance clinicians' ability to detect problematic eating behaviors and to thoughtfully select among available treatment approaches for these more unusual cases.

Despite efforts to achieve greater diagnostic specificity by refining diagnostic criteria in the fifth edition of *Diagnostic and Statistical Manual for Mental Disorders* (DSM-5, American Psychiatric Association 2013), a large proportion of patients who present with eating-related concerns display "atypical presentations" or have symptoms that meet criteria for other specified feeding or eating disorder (OSFED) or unspecified feeding or eating disorder (UFED). In atypical presentations, symptoms may appear less intense: patients may report low frequency of binge eating/purging and present at a normal body mass index (BMI); patients may present primarily with somatic symptoms (e.g., rumination, eating nonnutritive substances, etc.), and patients may deny body image concerns (e.g., avoidant and restrictive food intake disorder). Clinicians may therefore find themselves unsure as to how to classify and treat these patients. This may result in underdetection and undertreatment. Yet, patients with atypical presentations, including OSFED and UFED, still display clinically significant distress and/or impairment in functioning, in turn increasing the likelihood of psychological and physical sequelae. To enhance provision of effective treatment, this chapter aims to increase clinician's awareness of these presentations. Because avoidant/restrictive food intake disorder (ARFID) is discussed elsewhere in this book (see Chapter 5), it is not explicitly addressed here.

Key Diagnostic Checklist

❏ *Pica:* The ingestion of a substance with no substantial nutritional value on a regular basis over a period of at least 1 month.

❏ *Rumination disorder:* A disorder characterized by frequent and repeated swallowing and regurgitation of food into the mouth for a period of at least 1 month without the presence of nausea or involuntary vomiting.

❏ *Other specified feeding or eating disorder: A diagnosis* warranted when a patient presents with feeding or eating behaviors that result in a significant distress and/or impairment in areas of functioning (e.g., relationships, work, self-care, health) but do not meet the full criteria for any of the other feeding and eating disorders; OSFED includes atypical anorexia nervosa, subthreshold binge-eating disorder, subthreshold bulimia nervosa, purging disorder, and night eating syndrome.

Diagnostic Rule Outs

Medical

- Thyroid problems that could affect appetite and/or weight
- Other medical problems that might explain symptoms (e.g., cancer, esophageal reflux, ulcer, brain tumor)
- Medications that could affect appetite and/or weight, such as stimulant medications for attention-deficit disorder
- Nutrient absorption deficiencies
- General overeating (in contrast to binge eating characterized by a loss of control)

Psychiatric

- Depression—weight loss or gain secondary to depressed mood

- Psychosis
- Physical or emotional neglect or abuse

Epidemiology and Risk Factors

Epidemiology

- *Pica.* Prevalence estimates for pica vary. Among individuals with developmental delays/disabilities, estimates range from 0.3% to 25.8% (Ali 2001; Ashworth et al. 2008). Observed rates of pica appear to be particularly high in pregnant women in developing countries (up to 74%) (Ngozi 2008).
- *Rumination disorder.* Prevalence estimates for rumination disorder vary. Higher prevalence in individuals with developmental disabilities (6%–10%) have been reported (Olden 2001).
- *OSFED.* In community samples, prevalence of OSFED is estimated to be around 5% in adolescent samples, with similar impairment levels as full those meeting full diagnostic criteria for an eating disorder. In one study, observed 3-month prevalence rates for older adolescents and adults were 0.7% for subthreshold bulimia nervosa, 6.92% for binge-eating disorder subthresholds, and 0.58% for purging disorder. Up to 25% of patients presenting for treatment have symptoms that appear to meet criteria for OSFED (Fairweather-Schmidt and Wade 2014; Mancuso et al. 2015; Wade and O'Shea 2015).

Risk Factors

- *Pica.* This disorder is more common among adults with intellectual disabilities or another mental disorder and during pregnancy and may be experienced as specific craving for a nonfood substance
- *Rumination disorder.* Rumination appears more commonly among individuals with developmental disabilities (up to 10%; Gravestock 2000) and in those with other eating concerns (Delaney et al. 2015).
- *OSFED.* Risk factors for OSFED are the same as those associated with onset of full syndrome disorders of anorexia nervosa, binge-eating disorder, and bulimia nervosa

Common Comorbidities

Medical

- *Pica.* Common risks associated with pica include chocking, ingesting harmful or life-threatening materials or objects that may require surgical removal, and death (Stiegler 2005; Matson et al. 2013).

- *Rumination disorder.* Rumination may result in weight loss (in up to 40% of patients) and malnutrition, particularly if it occurs immediately after eating or is accompanied by restriction of food intake, as some individuals may avoid eating to avoid displaying this behavior in social situations (Nicholls and Bryant-Waugh 2009); dental erosions; and halitosis; as well as electrolyte abnormalities (Absah et al. 2017).

- *OSFED.* Medical concerns related to atypical and subthreshold disorders include atypical anorexia nervosa (AN) (medical causes of weight loss and medical consequences of malnutrition), bulimia nervosa (BN) (including electrolyte abnormalities, cardiac problems, dental caries, esophageal tears), binge-eating disorder (BED), purging (similar to BN), and night eating syndrome (similar to overweight and obesity, including diabetes and hypertension).

Psychiatric

- *Pica.* Individuals with developmental delays/disabilities, autism spectrum disorder.

- *Rumination disorder.* individuals with developmental disabilities and eating disorders.

- *OSFED.* Depression, anxiety disorders, obsessive-compulsive disorder, autism spectrum disorder.

Clinical Presentations

Case 1: Noah (Pica)

Noah is a 12-year-old with intellectual disability. Parents reported that he ingests napkins and other paper products when there are changes to his routines—for example, when his father leaves on a business trip or when he has to transition to new environments. Parents noted that Noah appears anxious and agitated in these situations, clenching and unclenching his fists and scanning the room before grabbing napkins, tissues, and other paper products.

Case 2: Jane (Rumination Disorder)

Jane is a 23-year-old female presenting with obesity, binge eating, and rumination. Jane endorsed experiencing effortless regurgitation without any gagging. Jane noted that food would come up back into her mouth within an hour of eating food. She identified rumination as initial focus of treatment. Jane reports a lifelong history of regurgitating foods. With self-monitoring, Jane was able to identify that regurgitation (and binge eating) would most frequently occur in the evenings, if she is doing work. According to Jane, she would ruminate only after "normal" eating episodes, eliminating binge eating as trigger for rumination. Jane noted that she would spit out food in the evenings. Jane also recorded instances of regurgitation at work but noted that these are less noticeable because she swallows the food back and covers her mouth rather than spitting.

Case 3: John (Other Specified Feeding or Eating Disorder [Atypical Anorexia Nervosa])

John is a 19-year-old male who was previously overweight. John began changing his eating behaviors during his freshman year of college after being told by his primary care physician that his BMI was in the overweight range. John became concerned with improving his athletic performance; he reduced his carbohydrate intake, eliminated desserts and fast food, and began working out on a daily basis, doing a combination of cardiovascular exercise and weightlifting. John also described eating large volumes of green vegetables at every meal and worrying about not "getting enough" lean proteins. John lost 35 pounds in the span of 3 months, although his BMI remained in the normal weight. At intake he presented with signs of malnutrition, including difficulty concentrating, being cold and tired all the time, spending a lot of time reading fitness blogs and research recipes, and having a low sex drive. John reported wanting to be "ripped."

Assessment

Pica and rumination disorder can be assessed using the Pica, ARFID, Rumination Disorder Interview (PARDI; Bryant-

Waugh and Cooke 2017). Questions from both measures aim to facilitate diagnosis of the aforementioned conditions based on DSM-5 criteria and allow for specification of frequency (how often the behavior is occurring) and severity in terms of avoidance and/or impairment in social situations and medical sequelae (Bryant-Waugh and Cooke 2017).

The PARDI can be used to assess presence and severity of rumination, helping the assessor to differentiate between rumination disorder and other eating related concerns (e.g., vomiting, BN, gastroesophageal reflux disease [GERD]). In rumination disorder, regurgitation does not serve the function of getting rid of calories. The regurgitation typically occurs spontaneously, less than an hour after eating, and occurs in waves versus all in once. Small amounts of foods will come up repeatedly after an eating episode (Tucker et al. 2013). Content typically contains food pieces that the patient recently ingested and does not have an acidic aftertaste. Many patients deny nausea or pain before rumination occur, but those features may be present.

Evidence-Based Treatments (All Level 4, Experimental)

Pica

Treatment depends on presumed etiology. If a nutritional/ mineral deficiency is suspected, it will be treated first via nutritional supplements. If a behavioral etiology is assumed, a functional assessment should be conducted. If the behavior appears to be rooted in learning contingencies (e.g., attention, stimulation), then treatment should be more behavioral in nature, addressing sensory, automatic, or other reinforcement contingencies. In individuals with developmental delays, treatment focuses on identifying conditions under which behavior occurs, as well as functions of behavior (e.g., self-soothing, attention). For individuals with intellectual disabilities, strategies for managing the environment by removing foods that trigger the behavior or contingencies that maintain behavior, such as staff attention, have been described.

Rumination Disorder

No treatment for rumination disorder has been systematically studied and received extensive empirical scrutiny and support. Evidence from case studies and theoretical reports suggests that, across all patient populations, treatment is behavioral. Diaphragmatic breathing as a form of habit reversal strategy appears to be particularly beneficial. Cognitive-behavioral therapy (CBT) has also been proposed to treat rumination in adults.

OSFED

Treatments for OSFED are typically those offered for the full-syndrome condition (Figure 6–1): atypical anorexia nervosa in adolescents (family-based treatment [FBT], systemic family therapy, CBT); atypical anorexia nervosa in adults (CBT); binge-eating disorder (CBT, dialectical behavioral therapy, behavioral weight management); bulimia nervosa (FBT or CBT for adolescents; CBT or interpersonal psychotherapy for adults); ARFID (FBT or CBT); and night eating syndrome (strategies informed by CBT).

Treatments for Atypical Clinical Syndromes

Pica

Pica is defined as the ingestion of a substance with no substantial nutritional value on a regular basis over a period of at least 1 month. Examples of substances ingested include glass, ice, sharp objects, bodily fluids, hair, clay, paper and related products, and paint. Diagnostic criteria specify that the eating behavior is inappropriate given the developmental level of the individual and is not part of a culturally sanctioned practice. DSM-5 criteria also recommend a minimum age of 2 years for a pica diagnosis, to exclude developmentally normal mouthing of objects by infants that sometimes results in ingestion. If the behavior occurs in the context of another condition, such as intellectual/developmental delays, schizophrenia, or pregnancy, the condition may warrant a separate diagnosis when it requires separate treatment.

Common risks associated with pica include choking, ingestion of harmful or life-threatening materials or objects that may require surgical removal, and death (Matson et al. 2013; Stiegler 2005). Although childhood onset is most common, pica can occur across the life span. In adulthood, the condition is particularly common among adults with intellectual

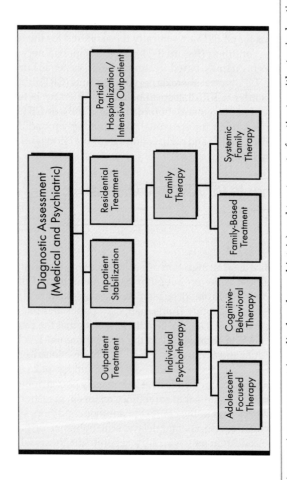

FIGURE 6–1. Diagnostic assessment (medical and psychiatric) and treatment of patients with atypical eating presentations.

disabilities or another mental disorder. Pica may also present during pregnancy and be experienced as specific craving for a nonfood substance.

Prevalence estimates for pica vary. Among individuals with developmental delays/disabilities, estimates range from 0.3% to 25.8% (Ali 2001; Ashworth et al. 2008). Observed rates of pica appear to be particularly high in pregnant women in developing countries—up to 74% (Ngozi 2008).

Research regarding etiology of pica is limited. In general cases pica can be attributed to 1) mineral deficiency (e.g., iron), such that the individual is eating an object containing the mineral that they are missing; 2) obsessive-compulsive spectrum disorder (Hergüner et al. 2008); or 3) sensory, physiological, or social consequences of eating. In particular, for individuals with developmental delays, pica may provide stimulation, satisfy a "sensory craving," or draw the attention of others.

Treatment depends on the presumed etiology. If a nutritional/mineral deficiency is suspected, it will be treated first via nutritional supplements, such as in the case of pregnancy. If the behavior appears to be rooted in learning contingencies (i.e., attention, stimulation), then treatment should be more behavioral in nature, addressing sensory, automatic, or other reinforcement contingencies. For example, if attention from others appears to motivate behavior, then the eating behavior will be ignored. Indeed, in individuals with developmental delays, treatment focuses on identifying conditions under which the behavior occurs as well as functions of behavior (e.g., self-soothing, attention) (Hagopian and Adelinis 2001; Kern et al. 2006). Subsequently, the item that stimulates pica behaviors is removed from the environment and/or alternative responses that serve a similar function or response blocking (i.e., stopping the behavior from taking place) are implemented and reinforced with rewards.

Rumination Disorder

Rumination disorder is characterized by frequent and repeated swallowing and regurgitation of food into the mouth for a period of at least 1 month without the presence of nausea or involuntary vomiting. The behavior occurs across the age spectrum (Soykan et al. 1997) and may have a lifelong course. In adults, rumination appears to co-occur among individuals with developmental disabilities (up to 10%; Gravestock 2000) and in those with other eating concerns (Delaney et al. 2015). The person may rechew and reswallow the food or spit it out. Whereas infants will present with stereotypical movements (i.e., arching the back with head held back and making sucking movements), older children and adults may attempt to disguise the behavior by placing a hand over their mouth, coughing, and swallowing. To avoid displaying this behavior in front of others due to social embarrassment, older children and adults may also avoid eating prior to or in social situations.

Rumination behaviors frequently occur within 10 minutes of finishing eating and last up to 2 hours; the regurgitate typically tastes similar to the food ingested and lacks the sour, bitter, or acidic taste associated with GERD or vomiting. Patients also rarely report nausea, pain, or heartburn. The regurgitated food may be rechewed, reswallowed, or spit out.

It is necessary to establish that regurgitation is not due to a medical condition and does not occur exclusively in the course of another eating disorder. Although rumination is more frequently reported in infants and people with developmental disabilities, it also occurs in children and adults of normal intelligence.

The pathophysiology of rumination entails activation of the abdominal wall to increase intragastric pressure, which in turns leads to regurgitation of food that the patient has recently eaten. Until recently, rumination syndrome was diagnosed based on symptoms after ruling out structural abnormalities. More recently, it has been suggested that rumination can be diagnosed via high resolution or gastroduodenal manometry.

If another mental disorder, such as intellectual developmental disorder or psychotic spectrum disorder are present, rumination should be severe enough to warrant separate intervention.

Rumination may result in weight loss (in up to 40% of patients) and malnutrition—particularly if it occurs immediately after eating or is accompanied by restriction of food intake, as some may avoid eating to avoid displaying this behavior in social situations (Nicholls and Bryant-Waugh 2009)—dental erosions, halitosis, and electrolyte abnormalities (Absah et al. 2017).

No treatment for rumination disorder has been systematically studied or received extensive empirical scrutiny and support. Evidence from case studies and theoretical reports suggest that across all patient populations, effective treatment is behavioral in nature. Treatment frequently focuses on education about rumination and pathophysiology underlying this behavior, self-monitoring to identify triggers. The use of habit reversal involves teaching an incompatible behavior (diaphragmatic breathing). For children, social support from the patient's parents is usually needed. For individuals with intellectual disabilities, strategies for managing the environment by removing foods that trigger the behavior or contingencies that maintain behavior, such as increased attention, have been described.

Recently, Thomas and Murray (2016) proposed a cognitive-behavioral formulation and treatment of rumination focusing on processes that maintain rumination behavior once it is formed. Consistent with other treatment approaches, rumination is conceptualized as a habit. Contraction of the abdominal wall after eating causes an urge that leads to the opening of the esophageal sphincter, which facilitates regurgitation of food. The authors propose that internal triggers (emotions such as disgust, shame, and anxiety and physical sensations such as fullness), as well as external cues (types/quantities of food, time of the day, triggers that activate body image concerns), may amplify this urge and thus negatively reinforce this behavior in some patients because the behavior provides relief. Accordingly, intervention includes

1. Providing patients with psychoeducation about symptoms, etiology of rumination, potential medical (e.g., malnutrition, tooth decay, choking, aspiration) and social consequences, as well as putative maintenance factors.
2. Self-monitoring of rumination episodes to identify triggers for rumination (e.g., time of day; internal states such as emotions and physiological sensations that are more likely to trigger rumination; environmental cues, such as types of food eaten, places, people, and circumstances). Patients are asked to record every episode, note the context in which the episode occurred (time of the day; events preceding rumination, including eating episodes). A key component of self-monitoring is to increase awareness and sense of self-efficacy by helping patients and families identify the triggers for rumination. Many patients and families seek a medical explanation for their symptoms; thus, it is essential to help identify patient behaviors that promote regurgitation.

3. Diaphragmatic breathing training, which restores the gastroesophageal pressure and thus prevents rumination. Patients are taught *diaphragmatic breathing*—breathing slowly "in and out" such that the chest is motionless while the abdomen falls as the patient inhales and rises as the patient exhales, with each breath lasting at least 3 seconds. Patients are instructed to practice diaphragmatic breathing after each meal and are also encouraged to practice diaphragmatic breathing on a regular basis, such as after episodes of rumination, at set times, or during periods of physical activity. Results to date support the efficacy of diaphragmatic breathing performed alone or combined with other therapies.

4. Patient-specific strategies that are based on the individual cognitive-behavioral formulation and relapse prevention. For example, patients may be taught to identify and address unhelpful thought patterns that increase anxiety. Patients may also be taught be taught assertiveness skills to manage challenging interpersonal interactions that may trigger anxiety, and subsequently urges.

Other Specified Feeding or Eating Disorder

Based on DSM-5 criteria, a diagnosis of OSFED is warranted when a patient presents with feeding or eating behaviors that result in a significant distress and/or impairment in areas of functioning (e.g., relationships, work, self-care, health) but do not meet the full criteria for any of the other feeding and eating disorders. As noted earlier, because patients have atypical presentations in which symptoms may appear less intense (i.e., patients may report low frequency of binge eating/purging, present at a normal BMI, and/or present primarily with somatic symptoms [e.g., rumination] while denying body image concerns), clinicians may find themselves unsure as to how to classify and treat these patients. This may result in underdetection and undertreatment.

The diagnostic label will frequently spell out why the person's presentation did not meet criteria for another eating disorder. OSFED presentations include the following:

- *Atypical anorexia nervosa.* All criteria for AN are met, except despite significant weight loss, the individual's weight is within or above the normal range. Frequently individuals with this presentation were at higher weight or overweight prior to initiating dieting efforts. Preliminary research suggests that patients presenting with as little as 5% or 10% weight loss and eating behaviors and cognitions characteristic of AN will display elevated eating pathology and distress relative to control participants (Forney et al. 2017). What is concerning is that despite distress, greater degree of weight loss, high functional impairment, and sequelae of malnutrition, patients with a history of overweight/obesity are less likely to receive inpatient medical care relative to patients with AN without history of overweight/obesity (Kennedy et al. 2017).

- *Bulimia nervosa of low frequency and/or limited duration.* All of the criteria for BN are met except that the binge eating and inappropriate compensatory behavior occur at a lower frequency and/or for less than 3 months.

- *Binge-eating disorder of low frequency and/or limited duration.* All of the criteria for BED are met, except at a lower frequency and/or for less duration than required for full-syndrome BED.

- *Purging disorder.* The individual exhibits recurrent purging behavior to influence weight or shape in the absence of binge eating.

- *Night eating syndrome (NES).* The individual has recurrent episodes of night eating, as manifested by eating after awakening from sleep or by excessive food consumption after the evening meal. The behavior causes significant distress/impairment and is not better explained by environmental influences or social norms or by another mental health disorder (e.g., BED).

Data on etiology of OSFED are limited. Clinical experience suggests that OSFED presentations do not significantly differ in course and response to treatment from full-syndrome eating disorders. Clinical considerations include fear of excess weight gain, which at times may be more intense in individuals with atypical AN, as some of these patients were overweight at baseline and thus are extremely fearful of that outcome.

Atypical Anorexia Nervosa

Among adolescents with AN, FBT has extensive empirical support (Lock 2010, 2015). As discussed elsewhere (see Chapter 2), treatment entails empowering parents to facilitate renourishment efforts. A similar approach can be adopted for the treatment of children and adolescents with atypical AN. Emphasis should be placed on psychological, physiological, and social effects of malnutrition and restrictive eating patterns. Despite their seemingly "normal" weight, children and adolescents with atypical AN frequently present with signs of malnutrition secondary to caloric restriction and weight loss. Individuals presenting with eating disorders of limited duration may respond more favorably to treatment, because their eating challenges are not firmly rooted.

Purging Disorder

Data on epidemiology, etiology, and treatment of purging disorder are scarce. Lifetime prevalence estimates for purging disorder vary from 1.1% (Favaro et al. 2003) to 5.3% (Wade et al. 2006). Whereas some studies suggest that individuals with purging disorder report lower levels of comorbid psychopathology, eating disorder psychopathology, and higher self-esteem then those with BN, other studies find that persons with purging disorder do not significantly differ from those with BN in terms of symptoms severity, body dissatisfaction, and dietary restraint (Binford and Le Grange 2005; Keel and Haedt 2008; Keel et al. 2001, 2005). A recent meta-analysis by Smith et al. (2017) of 38 studies comparing purging disorder with DSM-5 eating disorders (i.e., AN, BN, BED) and non–eating disorder control subjects concluded that purging disorder is associated with later age at onset (relative to AN and BN), shorter course of illness (relative to BED), and better prognosis (relative to other eating disorders). Moreover, persons with purging disorder appear to display lower levels of impulsivity, perfectionism, body dissatisfaction, and levels of eating psychopathology, less frequent purging, and higher levels of self-esteem than those with symptoms meeting diagnostic criteria for BN.

Although lack of objective binge-eating episodes may contribute to less frequent purging in purging disorder, individuals may still present with physical complications similar to those observed in patients with BN. Indeed, some preliminary data suggest that purging disorder is associated with a higher mortality ratio than that observed in BN and AN purging subtypes (Koch et al. 2013, 2014).

Clinically, individuals with purging disorder frequently also display heightened sensitivity to sensations of fullness.

Moreover, a pattern of frequent vomiting after regular-sized meals may be more challenging to eradicate, and thus degree of subjective loss of control would be important to assess. Although the evidence base is lacking, individuals with purging disorder may benefit from empirically supported interventions for BN (Knott et al. 2015; Sysko and Hildebrandt 2011).

Night Eating Syndrome

Clinically, individuals with NES also frequently present with low appetite in the morning, fewer eating episodes during the day than non-NES individuals, a strong urge to eat in the evening, the belief that one needs to eat to fall asleep, and depressed mood during the day that appears to worsen by evening hours (Allison et al. 2005, 2010b). NES may co-occur with another eating disorder. Up to a quarter of individuals with NES have symptoms that also meet criteria for BED, and approximately 9% of individuals with BN are also estimated to have NES.

Case studies provide preliminary support for use of progressive muscle relaxation techniques, behavioral weight loss, and CBT adapted for NES to reduce occurrence of night eating (Berner and Allison 2013). CBT for NES (Allison et al. 2010a) consists of ten 1-hour sessions. Patients are assigned self-monitoring to identify circumstances under which night eating occurs and to help patients reflect on their eating and sleep patterns. To facilitate this process, therapists teach patients behavioral chain analyses to identify intervention targets. Initial focus is on introducing environmental interventions to reduce nocturnal ingestion, such as placing signs on the fridge to remind patients of their intentions and having patients create a pros and cons of night eating card for them to review before bed. Stimulus control strategies may also focus on availability of food and access to food during the night. Patients are also taught strategies to regulate eating during the day, increasing the frequency of eating episodes. Weight loss and improved sleep hygiene may also be identified as goals of treatment. Thus, elements from CBT for insomnia are incorporated as appropriate. In the second phase of treatment, cognitive strategies are taught to address problematic thinking patterns, including those related to sleep (i.e., the need to eat in order to fall asleep) and those more broadly maintaining depression. Behavioral strategies are used to facilitate sleep hygiene, improve stress management (e.g., progressive muscle relaxation, physical activity), and regulate eating (e.g., adding breakfast). The last phase (two sessions) is focused on reviewing progress and relapse prevention.

Treatments Illustrated

Pica (Behavioral Therapy; see Case 1)

For Noah, the 12-year-boy with intellectual disability who ingested paper products presented earlier, a behavioral approach was adopted. Parents were encouraged to observe Noah to identify circumstances under which ingestion of paper products occurs. The goal was to identify triggers for anxiety (cues) and introduce alternative coping mechanisms. Noah's parents were encouraged to present a daily schedule to Noah, orient him to upcoming transitions, and scaffold use of alternative self-soothing skills, such as hugging his favorite stuffed animal. They were encouraged to verbally praise use of alternative coping strategies, offering soothing when appropriate without reinforcing problem behavior. As part of self-monitoring, Noah's parents were taught to recognize early signs of anxiety in Noah. For example, they noticed that Noah would start frowning and that his body become rigid when he became anxious. To facilitate Noah's ability to self-monitor, the parents were instructed to notice times when Noah would start displaying physical symptoms of anxiety and verbalize this for Noah. The parents and Noah were also taught a child-adapted version of progressive muscle relaxation. To help Noah practice use of skills, parents created a sticker chart that they put in Noah's room. The parents were instructed to help Noah practice progressive relaxation skills three times a day (in the morning, after school, and in the evening) by modeling and providing step-by-step guidance. Earning two out of three stickers would earn Noah a small reward at the end of the day as well as praise for the parents. Subsequently, both in the presence of anxiety triggers and when Noah would display physical symptoms of anxiety, Noah's parents would model and scaffold Noah's use of diaphragmatic breathing or progressive relaxation skills. After several weeks, with coaching from his parents, Noah displayed good use of alternative self-soothing skills and progressive relaxation skills when feeling anxious.

To facilitate differential reinforcement, the therapist also instructed Noah's parents in the use of exposure procedures. Whereas initially Noah's parents tried to limit his access to paper products, particularly around transition times, they gradually started to reintroduce paper products. For example, when Noah arrived home from school, he would have an afternoon snack. In the past, Noah would frequently become restless as the snack was being prepared and served and would try to put a paper napkin in his mouth. Once Noah displayed good mastery of alternative strategies, a paper napkin was placed on the table along with his snack. Noah was reminded that he should eat his snack and that the paper napkin was not for eating. He was instructed by his mother to take a few deep breaths and to start eating his snack.

Noah's parents found that they initially had more success when alternatives to paper products were highly reinforcing. In Noah's case the parents had good success redirecting Noah when he was presented with peanut butter and crackers for his afternoon snack. Noah was also praised for eating the snack and not grabbing the paper napkin. When at first Noah tried to grab the paper napkin, he was gently redirected to eating the snack, such that his mother placed Noah's hands on the snack, taking the paper napkin out of his hands while speaking in a soothing voice and prompting Noah to start eating his snack. The procedure was repeated over several days and also at other times during the day. Over time, the parents reported that Noah stopped trying to grab the paper napkin. Noah's parents were able to fade out coaching, with Noah independently eating his snack or using self-soothing skills. By treatment end, pica behavior stopped altogether, although around unexpected transitions Noah still needed a reminder and at times some coaching from his parents to use alternative skills.

Rumination Disorder (Cognitive-Behavioral Therapy; see Case 2)

The therapist working with Jane, the 23-year-old female presenting with obesity, binge eating, and rumination discussed earlier, adopted a cognitive-behavioral framework based on Thomas and Murray's (2016) work. During the first phase of treatment, Jane was provided with psychoeducation about the pathophysiology of rumination as well as potential complications. This discussion appeared to reduce Jane's feelings of shame and self-blame. Jane also shared that she was very concerned about displaying these behaviors at work, noting that she avoids eating lunch with colleagues or going out to eat with friends as a result. Jane also expressed concern about dating. She expressed worrying about being able to date because a potential partner would find rumination disgusting. Self-monitoring was introduced

next. Jane was asked to write down time and number of regurgitation episodes.

The therapist and Jane reviewed self-monitoring records
at next session. Jane appeared to benefit from self-monitoring, as she was able to link environmental triggers (increasing demands at work, conflict with parents, down mood)
and feeling anxious to both rumination and binge eating.
Jane also noted that regurgitation was more likely to take
place when she ate quickly or ate certain foods, particularly
pasta and milk. Jane reported that she would sometimes spit
the food and sometimes would swallow it. She acknowledged
that she liked the taste of regurgitated food and thus would
prefer to reswallow it. At the same time, she endorsed a
strong desire to lose weight and reported that being able to
spit food out "felt like a free pass to eat what I like."

At the next session the therapist introduced diaphragmatic breathing as a habit reversal strategy. The therapist
demonstrated and modeled use of diaphragmatic breathing
in session. Jane was also asked to practice diaphragmatic
breathing in session with therapist providing corrective
feedback, asking Jane to slow down her pace to allow at least
3 seconds for each inhalation and exhalation. Jane was asked
to practice diaphragmatic breathing multiple times per day,
particularly during times that were identified as high risk
for rumination. She was asked to practice before, during,
and at regular intervals in the hour subsequent to eating dinner. Subsequently, Jane's triggers and diaphragmatic breathing were added to the self-monitoring record. Jane reported
that she found learning diaphragmatic breathing very helpful for addressing rumination. Jane was instructed to slowly
chew her food at meals and practice diaphragmatic breathing
after meals for at least 10–20 minutes.

Jane also found it helpful to engage in alternative behaviors after meals, such as talking to colleagues or watching
funny animal videos on her phone. To address residual
rumination episodes, the therapist and Jane focused on addressing mood regulation functions of rumination. Jane
benefited from behavioral activation to improve mood (e.g.,
going for walks, making plans with friends, going to movies)
and learning assertiveness skills to set boundaries at work
and with parents.

To address weight and shape concerns, the therapist
and Jane tracked her weight on a weight graph to test Jane's
belief that her weight would increase drastically if she were
to stop ruminating. Over the course of treatment, Jane observed that despite week to week fluctuations, her weight
essentially remained the same. Although binge eating was
not a direct focus of treatment, Jane reported that frequency

of binge eating episodes had drastically decreased over the course of treatment.

By the end of treatment Jane was no longer experiencing rumination and endorsed having one subjective binge eating episode in the week prior to treatment termination. The last session focused on relapse prevention. Jane was encouraged to start fading out diaphragmatic breathing, using it primarily when she noticed she had the urge to ruminate or when feeling physical symptoms of anxiety. The therapist and Jane also made a list of triggers for rumination/binge eating along with strategies that Jane found helpful.

Other Specified Feeding or Eating Disorder (Cognitive-Behavioral Therapy for Atypical Anorexia Nervosa; see Case 3)

John, the 19-year-old male discussed earlier who had been overweight but had developed eating and exercise behaviors and choices that led to malnutrition, was oriented to enhanced CBT (CBT-E) and phases of treatment. The first phase of treatment focused on psychoeducation and real-time self-monitoring. John was provided with extensive psychoeducation about the physical, psychological, and cognitive sequelae of undereating and malnutrition. John also discussed the social ramifications of dieting. He reported that he stopped going to the dining hall or spending time with friends. John also stated that although he did well academically and passed all of his exams, he could not recall much of what he learned. John responded well to CBT-E, with first goal of treatment being renourishment and normalization of eating patterns. John found real time self-monitoring helpful to for identifying and addressing problematic eating patterns. For example, John observed that he would become very hungry in the early afternoon, which would lead to extreme irritability and low energy. John also observed that he would be most comfortable eating prepackaged food, because he would feel reassured by knowing the caloric content of what he was eating. A focus of treatment was on addressing fears around John becoming overweight and helping John incorporate energy-dense foods in a more balanced manner.

Treatment also focused on helping John redistribute intake more equally through the day as he tended to "hoard" his calories because he feared he would get "too hungry" at night. For example, John found that he benefited from having two afternoon snacks. This helped to address moodiness in the afternoon and hunger later in the evening. Toward the middle of treatment, the therapist and John helped John to learn to monitor and respond appropriately to hunger and fullness cues. John was able to identify anchors on his "hunger" and "fullness" scale to prompt John starting and stopping eating. The later stage of treatment focused on helping John transition to going back to college, including learning how to eat in the college cafeteria, navigating social challenges, and balancing academics with other priorities. At the end of treatment, John reported that he found the language of "building healthy habits" particularly helpful. John also shared with the therapist that early on in treatment he found the therapist providing reassurance and encouraging John to increase variety as "reassuring."

Common Outcomes and Complications

- Pica

  - Behavioral interventions can lead to cessation of ingestion behavior.

  - Continued ingestion of nonnutritive items may lead to malnutrition or poisoning, including lead poisoning, or damage to organs.

- Rumination disorder

  - Case studies suggest that CBT-informed intervention facilitates cessation of rumination.

  - Adverse outcomes may include enamel erosion, malnutrition, and complications similar to those seen in bulimia nervosa.

- Other specified feeding or eating disorder

  - Patients appear to benefit from the same evidence-based treatments used for full-threshold disorders.

  - The physical, psychological, cognitive, and social impairments are similar to those in full-syndrome disorders

Resources and Further Reading

Training Resources

CBT: Oxford Cognitive Therapy Centre: https://www.octc.co.uk/training

FBT: Training Institute for Child and Adolescent Eating Disorders: train2treat4ed.com

Fairburn CG: Cognitive Behavioral Therapy and Eating Disorders. New York, Guilford, 2008

Lock J, Le Grange D: Treatment Manual for Anorexia Nervosa: A Family Based Approach, 2nd Edition. New York, Guilford, 2013

Murphy R, Straebler S, Cooper Z, et al: Interpersonal psychotherapy (IPT) for the treatment of eating disorders, in Evidence Based Treatments for Eating Disorders. Edited by Dancyger IF, Fornari V. New York, Nova, 2009, pp 257–275

Safer DL, Telch CF, Chen EY: Dialectical Behavior Therapy for Binge Eating and Bulimia. New York, Guilford, 2009

Further Reading

Pica

National Eating Disorders Association: https://www.nationaleatingdisorders.org/learn/by-eating-disorder/other/pica

Delaney CB, Eddy KT, Hartmann AS, et al: Pica and rumination behavior among individuals seeking treatment for eating disorders or obesity. Int J Eat Disord 48(2):238–248, 2015

Mishori R, McHale C: Pica: an age-old eating disorder that's often missed. J Fam Pract 63(7):E1–E4, 2014

Rumination Disorder

Absah I, Rishi A, Talley NJ, et al: Rumination syndrome: pathophysiology, diagnosis, and treatment. Neurogastroenterol Motil Apr 29(4), 2017

Thomas JJ, Murray HB: Cognitive-behavioral treatment of adult rumination behavior in the setting of disordered eating: a single case experimental design. Int J Eat Disord 49(10):967–972, 2016

Other Specified Feeding or Eating Disorder

Berner LA, Allison KC: Behavioral management of night eating disorders. Psychol Res Behav Manag 6:1–8, 2013

Fairweather-Schmidt AK, Wade TD: DSM-5 eating disorders and other specified eating and feeding disorders: is there a meaningful differentiation? Int J Eat Disord 47(5):524–533, 2014

References

Absah I, Rishi A, Talley NJ, et al: Rumination syndrome: pathophysiology, diagnosis, and treatment. Neurogastroenterol Motil Apr 29(4), 2017 27766723

Ali Z: Pica in people with intellectual disability: a literature review of aetiology, epidemiology and complications. J Intellect Dev Disabil 26(3):205–215, 2001

Allison KC, Grilo CM, Masheb RM, et al: Binge eating disorder and night eating syndrome: a comparative study of disordered eating. J Consult Clin Psychol 73(6):1107–1115, 2005 16392984

Allison KC, Lundgren JD, Moore RH, et al: Cognitive behavior therapy for night eating syndrome: a pilot study. Am J Psychother 64(1):91–106, 2010a 20405767

Allison KC, Lundgren JD, O'Reardon JP, et al: Proposed diagnostic criteria for night eating syndrome. Int J Eat Disord 43(3):241–247, 2010b 19378289

American Psychiatric Association: Diagnostic and Statistical Manual of Mental Disorders, 5th Edition. Arlington, VA, American Psychiatric Association, 2013

Ashworth M, Martin L, Hirdes JP: Prevalence and correlates of pica among adults with intellectual disability in institutions. J Ment Health Res Intellect Disabil 1(3):176–190, 2008

Berner LA, Allison KC: Behavioral management of night eating disorders. Psychol Res Behav Manag 6:1–8, 2013 23569400

Binford RB, Le Grange D: Adolescents with bulimia nervosa and eating disorder not otherwise specified-purging only. Int J Eat Disord 38(2):157–161, 2005 16134105

Bryant-Waugh R, Cooke L: Poster presentation abstracts: 96 Development of the PARDI (Pica, ARFID, Rumination Disorder Interview): a structured assessment measure and diagnostic tool for feeding disorders. Arch Dis Child 102(suppl 3):A29, 2017

Delaney CB, Eddy KT, Hartmann AS, et al: Pica and rumination behavior among individuals seeking treatment for eating disorders or obesity. Int J Eat Disord 48(2):238–248, 2015 24729045

Fairweather-Schmidt AK, Wade TD: DSM-5 eating disorders and other specified eating and feeding disorders: is there a meaningful differentiation? Int J Eat Disord 47(5):524–533, 2014 24616045

Favaro A, Ferrara S, Santonastaso P: The spectrum of eating disorders in young women: a prevalence study in a general population sample. Psychosom Med 65(4):701–708, 2003 12883125

Forney KJ, Brown TA, Holland-Carter LA, et al: Defining "significant weight loss" in atypical anorexia nervosa. Int J Eat Disord 50(8):952–962, 2017 28436084

Gravestock S: Eating disorders in adults with intellectual disability. J Intellect Disabil Res 44(Pt 6):625–637, 2000 11115017

Hagopian LP, Adelinis JD: Response blocking with and without redirection for the treatment of pica. J Appl Behav Anal 34(4):527–530, 2001 11800195

Hergüner S, Ozyildirim I, Tanidir C: Is Pica an eating disorder or an obsessive-compulsive spectrum disorder? Prog Neuropsychopharmacol Biol Psychiatry 32(8):2010–2011, 2008 18848964

Keel PK, Haedt A: Evidence-based psychosocial treatments for eating problems and eating disorders. J Clin Child Adolesc Psychol 37(1):39–61, 2008

Keel PK, Mayer SA, Harnden-Fischer JH: Importance of size in defining binge eating episodes in bulimia nervosa. Int J Eat Disord 29(3):294–301, 2001 11262508

Keel PK, Haedt A, Edler C: Purging disorder: an ominous variant of bulimia nervosa? Int J Eat Disord 38(3):191–199, 2005 16211629

Kennedy GA, Forman SF, Woods ER, et al: History of overweight/obesity as predictor of care received at 1-year follow-up in adolescents with anorexia nervosa or atypical anorexia nervosa. J Adolesc Health 60(6):674–679, 2017 28284563

Kern L, Starosta K, Adelman B: Reducing pica by teaching children to exchange inedible items for edibles. Behav Modif 30(2):135–158, 2006 16464843

Knott S, Woodward D, Hoefkens A, et al: Cognitive behaviour therapy for bulimia nervosa and eating disorders not otherwise specified: translation from randomized controlled trial to a clinical setting. Behav Cogn Psychother 43(6):641–654, 2015 25331090

Koch S, Quadflieg N, Fichter M: Purging disorder: a comparison to established eating disorders with purging behaviour. Eur Eat Disord Rev 21(4):265–275, 2013 23629831

Koch S, Quadflieg N, Fichter M: Purging disorder: a pathway to death? A review of 11 cases. Eat Weight Disord 19(1):21–29, 2014 24198060

Lock J: Treatment of adolescent eating disorders: progress and challenges. Minerva Psichiatr 51(3):207–216, 2010 21532979

Lock J: An update on evidence-based psychosocial treatments for eating disorders in children and adolescents. J Clin Child Adolesc Psychol 44(5):707–721, 2015 25580937

Mancuso SG, Newton JR, Bosanac P, et al: Classification of eating disorders: comparison of relative prevalence rates using DSM-IV and DSM-5 criteria. Br J Psychiatry 206(6):519–520, 2015 25745131

Matson JL, Hattier MA, Belva B, et al: Pica in persons with developmental disabilities: approaches to treatment. Res Dev Disabil 34(9):2564–2571, 2013 23747942

Ngozi PO: Pica practices of pregnant women in Nairobi, Kenya. East Afr Med J 85(2):72–79, 2008 18557250

Nicholls D, Bryant-Waugh R: Eating disorders of infancy and childhood: definition, symptomatology, epidemiology, and comorbidity. Child Adolesc Psychiatr Clin N Am 18(1):17–30, 2009 19014855

Olden KW: Rumination. Curr Treat Options Gastroenterol 4(4):351–358, 2001 11469994

Smith KE, Crowther JH, Lavender JM: A review of purging disorder through meta-analysis. J Abnorm Psychol 126(5):565–592, 2017 28691846

Soykan I, Chen J, Kendall BJ, et al: The rumination syndrome: clinical and manometric profile, therapy, and long-term outcome. Dig Dis Sci 42(9):1866–1872, 1997 9331149

Stiegler LN: Understanding pica behavior: a review for clinical and education professionals. Focus Autism Other Dev Disabl 20(1):27–38, 2005

Sysko R, Hildebrandt T: Enhanced cognitive behavioural therapy for an adolescent with purging disorder: a case report. Eur Eat Disord Rev 19(1):37–45, 2011 20859990

Thomas JJ, Murray HB: Cognitive-behavioral treatment of adult rumination behavior in the setting of disordered eating: a single case experimental design. Int J Eat Disord 49(10):967–972, 2016 27302894

Tucker E, Knowles K, Wright J, Fox MR: Rumination variations: aetiology and classification of abnormal behavioural responses to digestive symptoms based on high-resolution manometry studies. Aliment Pharmacol Ther 37(2):263–274, 2013 23173868

Wade TD, Bergin JL, Tiggemann M, et al: Prevalence and long-term course of lifetime eating disorders in an adult Australian twin cohort. Aust N Z J Psychiatry 40(2):121–128, 2006 16476129

Wade TD, O'Shea A: DSM-5 unspecified feeding and eating disorders in adolescents: what do they look like and are they clinically significant? Int J Eat Disord 48(4):367–374, 2015 24854848

Chapter 7

Eating Disorders in the Context of Obesity

Cara Bohon, Ph.D.
Hannah Welch

Introduction

Despite common misperceptions, eating disorders occur in patients with comorbid medical obesity. Importantly, the intersection between obesity and eating disorders is not limited to binge-eating disorder (BED). Patients with obesity may also struggle with bulimia nervosa (BN), atypical anorexia nervosa (AN), or other eating disorders. This chapter provides tools and guidance for clinicians to recognize when an obese patient has a comorbid eating disorder and how to provide or recommend effective treatment.

Eating disorders currently recognized by DSM-5 (American Psychiatric Association 2013) can all occur in patients with obesity. Of note, DSM-5 removed absolute weight as a diagnostic criterion for AN, in part due to evidence of patients experiencing nearly all other symptoms of the disorder—both physical and psychological—at varying body mass index (BMI) levels. These patients still experience the debilitating effects of AN. Furthermore, DSM-5 introduced within the other specified feeding or eating disorder (OSFED) diagnosis the atypical AN presentation, in which all the criteria for AN are met except that the patient's weight, despite significant weight loss, is still within or above the normal range. Many of these patients were previously or are currently overweight or obese.

Research has shown a connection between obesity and BN (Fairburn et al. 2003). BN is characterized by a cycle of food restriction, binge eating, and compensatory behaviors. Distressed by their weight and hyperfocused on their body image, children with obesity are at risk of developing BN later in life (Fairburn et al. 2003). The cycle may begin when a patient restricts food intake to lose weight but then loses control and binge eats, followed by a compensatory behavior, such as purging, to eliminate calories consumed.

BED is the most common eating disorder in the context of obesity (Alexander et al. 2013). In 2014, 42% of patients with BED were obese, and among adults who were severely obese, up to 50% had been diagnosed with BED (Faulconbridge and Bechtel 2014). Despite high incidence rates of eating disorders in this population, physicians often acknowledge and focus on the weight specifically rather than the eating disorder and related behaviors—often exacerbating the latter.

Much as with AN, clinicians may expect that patients with avoidant/restrictive food intake disorder (ARFID) will be underweight. Nonetheless, low weight is not necessary for a diagnosis of ARFID. If a patient's ARFID is characterized by an extreme restriction—or even fear—of vegetables, for example, they can develop obesity because of overreliance on higher-calorie foods. Similarly, ARFID sometimes presents in children who will only eat a "beige diet" of high-carbohydrate and high-calorie foods, such as chicken nuggets, breads, and pasta, and as a result, they develop obesity early in life. Although there is little existing research on ARFID, clinical experience suggests considerable comorbidity between ARFID and obesity in patients who have presented with these patterns of behavior.

The greatest threat of an eating disorder in the context of obesity is that it will go undiagnosed and untreated. Despite increased education about eating disorders many people still equate disordered eating with low weight. When eating disorder symptoms are overlooked or, worse, praised as successful weight-loss behaviors, the disease will intensify and endure. This chapter provides clarity on how to prevent, diagnose, and treat eating disorders in the context of obesity.

Key Diagnostic Symptoms

Physical

❏ Severe weight loss over a short period of time—even if the patient is still medically overweight/obese or has a high body mass index. In cases of binge eating, weight gain may also be present.

❏ Hypotension and/or bradycardia—The patient's blood pressure and/or heart rate is low at rest.

❏ Orthostasis of blood pressure and/or heart rate—A large shift in blood pressure and/or heart rate when moving from supine to standing.

❏ Compensatory behaviors—Self-induced vomiting, excessive/compulsive exercise, compensatory fasting, or misuse of laxatives, diuretics, or diet pills.

❏ Electrolyte and vitamin imbalance, as well as decreased organ function.

Psychological

❏ Preoccupation with weight and shape—The patient spends a significant amount of time thinking about his/her weight (the number on the scale) and body shape, to the extent that it inhibits concentration at work or school and/or negatively affects interpersonal relationships and functioning.

❏ Food restriction—There is a dramatic reduction in overall food intake or certain food groups. Food rules are driven by fear of fats, fear of fatness, or fear of weight gain.

❏ Exercise compulsion—The patient exhibits driven or compelled exercise on a regular basis, where he/she becomes anxious if unable to carry out this obsession.

❏ Guilt and shame around eating—This can be an emotional response to binge eating (which includes a loss of control) or even to a normal meal after which the patient feels is excessive.

Diagnostic Rule Outs

Medical

• Thyroid problems that could affect appetite and/or weight

• Medications that could affect appetite and/or weight, such as stimulant medications for attention-deficit disorder

• Nutrient absorption deficiencies

• General overeating (in contrast to binge eating characterized by a loss of control)

Psychiatric

- Depression—weight loss or gain secondary to depressed mood

Epidemiology and Risk Factors

Epidemiology

- There is little research on the incidence of eating disorders in the context of obesity. Data from 2015 concluded that about 35% of Americans are obese, including 43% of Hispanics and 48% of non-Hispanic blacks (Hruby and Hu 2015). In general, lower socioeconomic status groups have higher rates of obesity (Hruby and Hu 2015). In addition, research has shown that more women are obese, regardless of their race, ethnicity, or socioeconomic status (Hruby and Hu 2015).

Risk Factors

- Improper guidance from medical team.
  - Clinicians often do not screen for an eating disorder when they see an obese patient and weight loss is praised even if achieved using maladaptive behaviors.
- Attention to the narrative around weight and shape.
  - Discussion of the obesity epidemic depicts patients as unhealthy and lazy, stigmatizing patients with obesity and driving some to adopt disordered eating (Andreyeva et al. 2008; Puhl and Suh 2015).
- Risk factors shared with eating disorders in the context of normal weight.
  - *Genetics.* Eating disorders run in families, and the risk of developing these disorders is even higher in the context of obesity (Thornton et al. 2011).
  - *Personality traits.* Personality traits increase risks for eating disorders and likely also do so in the context of obesity. These personality traits often among disorders; for example, patients with BN exhibit more impulsive tendencies than those with AN (Cassin and von Ranson 2005).

- *Disordered eating, dieting, and body image disturbance.* Abnormal behaviors include extreme dieting, skipping meals, eliminating certain foods or food groups completely, fasting, or creating and observing strict rules around eating.

Common Comorbidities

Medical

- *Diabetes.* Obesity is a major risk factor in developing diabetes, particularly type 2 diabetes (Citrome 2017).

- *Hypertension.* Obese individuals often have higher blood pressure due to an increase in fatty tissue around their heart and a subsequent stress on their arteries (Re 2009).

- *Cardiovascular disease.* Excess weight affects cholesterol in the body, and this makes patients more susceptible to heart disease and stroke (Lavie et al. 2009).

Psychiatric

- *Major depressive disorder.* Obesity increases the risk of developing depression and those who are depressed are at risk of developing obesity (Luppino et al. 2010).

- *Generalized anxiety disorder.* In one large sample, about two-thirds of people with eating disorders also had an anxiety disorder (Kaye et al. 2004).

- *Substance abuse.* Research has concluded that many eating disorder patients have comorbid substance abuse and should be considered when an eating disorder presents in the context of obesity (Holderness et al. 1994).

Clinical Presentations

Case 1: Maria (Atypical Anorexia in the Context of Obesity)

Maria is a 17-year-old Mexican American female with atypical anorexia nervosa. Maria presents for evaluation after

**losing more than 90 lb in 12 months secondary to severe
food restriction and excessive exercise.**

Her desire to lose weight began after a doctor noted that
her BMI of 37 was of concern because of health risks, such as
hypertension. She began eating what she considered to be a
"healthy" diet consisting entirely of salads. After losing an
initial 80 lb, she felt "stuck" at that weight and began decreasing her food intake even more. She began skipping entire meals and cutting out carbohydrates.

Maria denies binge eating, purging, or the use of laxatives
or diuretics to control her shape or weight, but she reports
exercising every day. She runs and/or does cardio exercise
on machines in the gym 40–60 minutes daily. Maria denies calorie counting but estimates eating no more than 1,200 calories
per day. She engages in "body checking" where she touches
body parts to make sure she has not gained weight. She weighs
herself daily, and if weight increases, she restricts food intake more that day. Higher weights also lead to greater anxiety throughout the day. Maria is 5'10" and weighs 175 lb at
evaluation. Her highest weight prior to the weight loss was
270 lb. Her food restriction leads to Maria feeling "tired all
the time" despite adequate sleep. She reports difficulty concentrating since her weight loss began and feels socially withdrawn. She isolates herself because so many social events
revolve around food. She denies symptoms of other psychiatric illnesses, such as poor mood or anxiety, aside from what
appears related to her eating disorder.

Case 2: Jason (Bulimia Nervosa in the Context of Obesity)

Jason is a 35-year-old white male with BED. Jason reports a
long history of binge eating, previously accompanied by
compensatory behaviors. He remembers being on diets
since age 8 or 9, which he believes led to an obsession about
food intake and shape/weight. He had a strong desire to
lose weight and tried many restrictive diets, eventually **engaging in binge eating and compensatory behaviors, including excessive exercise and food restriction.**

Jason reports that some days he is able to stay "on track"
and eat balanced and appropriate meals. However, on "bad
days" he will eat something "less healthy" for a meal, such
as a pasta with cream sauce and an accompanying dessert,
which then triggers continued "unhealthy" eating throughout the day. After a dinner of a burger and fries, he will
binge on a box of crackers with cheese. On these "bad days"
he notes that he **eats until he cannot eat anymore.** An addi-

tional example of a binge episode may be a package of cookies, two bars of chocolate, or a pint of ice cream.

Over the past couple of months before evaluation, he has ended every day with a binge-eating episode. However, he has not engaged in any compensatory behavior in 5–8 years. Jason reports that his mood is generally "ok" with some "typical stress."

Jason denies any other symptoms of psychiatric illness, although he does report history of depression. He denies history of drug use and currently drinks socially one or two glasses of wine per month.

Jason previously sought professional help with his eating as a child and again as a young adult. Therapy during college allowed him to cease his compensatory behaviors by focusing on health versus body shape. His symptoms are congruent with BED, including **daily binge episodes where he feels overly full, eats when he is not physically hungry, and feels consistently bad about his overeating.**

Case 3: Monica (Binge-Eating Disorder in the Context of Obesity)

Monica is a 20-year-old African American female with a 2-year history of BN. She began restricting food intake in attempt to lose weight after overhearing comments about her weight from peers on her dorm hall in college.

Monica has always been overweight or obese, as were most members of her family and her home community. Thus, she had never thought too much about her weight. She acknowledges that she feared for her mother's health because of a recent diagnosis of cardiac disease that the doctors believe to be related to her diet. After overhearing the comments from her peers, and also considering her mother's health, she decided to make some changes to her diet and try to lose weight. Monica tried to limit her food intake to 1,000 calories per day, as she had read that it would result in weight loss of 20 lb in 2 months. Despite this effort, she found herself turning to food whenever she was upset.

Starting college was a particularly stressful experience for Monica. She struggled to fit in and felt misunderstood by many of her peers who had grown up in different environments than she did. "Comfort foods" that reminded Monica of home, like cookies and ice cream that her family always had on hand, were often sought out after a difficult day.

After losing control and eating large quantities of these foods, she engaged in self-induced vomiting in order to get rid of those calories in attempt to stay below her 1,000-calorie daily intake target. Despite this effort, though, her weight continued to increase.

Eating Disorders in the Context of Obesity   **211**

Evidence-Based Outpatient Psychosocial Treatments for Eating Disorders in the Context of Obesity

Note: Studies of dialectical behavior therapy have included samples with high rates of obesity. Other studies may have included patients with obesity but did not explicitly study this population.

Adults

Cognitive-behavioral therapy (Fairburn et al. 2008)—Level 4 (experimental treatment)

Interpersonal psychotherapy (Agras et al. 2000)—Level 4 (experimental treatment)

Dialectical behavior therapy (Safer et al. 2001)—Level 1 (established treatment)

Children and Adolescents

Family-based treatment (Le Grange et al. 2015)—Level 4 (experimental treatment)

Cognitive-behavioral therapy (Fairburn et al. 2008)—Level 4 (experimental treatment)

Treatment Settings

Hospitalization for Medically Compromised Patients

Patients with an acute eating disorder in the context of obesity might require hospitalization. Damage to essential organs is possible when a patient has been restricting food intake for an extended period of time. In particular, muscles around the heart are affected by restriction, and this is manifested in a low heart rate (bradycardia). In addition, repetitive purging can cause an electrolyte imbalance that requires medical attention. Both of these behaviors can also cause orthostatic hypotension, which requires medical monitoring until vital signs normalize.

Residential Treatment

Residential treatment centers may be used as needed in follow-up to inpatient stay (although many patients transition from inpatient to outpatient care) and for cases in which patients do not respond to outpatient treatment. Importantly, there is no current evidence base supporting the efficacy of residential treatment programs (Frisch et al. 2006). Nevertheless, this can be an appropriate treatment option for a number of different cases: if patients were recently released from the hospital and needs a step down in care that cannot be provided in their home environment, if they are not medically compromised by their eating disorder but are at risk of hospitalization in the near future, or if they have been unresponsive to different outpatient treatment programs over an extended period of time. As mentioned, this can be an important treatment option for patients who have limited support in their recovery—whether they live alone, have a tumultuous home life, or something else. Residential programs give patients around-the-clock supervision and meal support, a cohort of other patients also in treatment, and therapy focused on eating disorders.

Partial Hospitalization

Partial hospital programs/intensive outpatient programs are for patients who might not be well suited for residential treatment but need more assistance around meals and lack family support for this purpose. These programs are a middle ground between the 24-hour care of residential treatment centers and outpatient therapy. They typically offer meal support for one or two meals and snacks per day, group therapy, and individual therapy multiple days per week.

Outpatient Therapy

Outpatient, evidence-based therapy is for patients whose quality of life has been disrupted by eating disturbances. This treatment option is suitable for patients who need professional help to alleviate eating disorder pathology and disturbances to psychosocial functioning. Specific options within this level of treatment include individual therapy with an eating disorder specialist (using cognitive-behavioral therapy [CBT], dialectical behavior therapy [DBT], or another evidence-based treatment), family therapy, and group therapy.

Medical Monitoring During Treatment

Regular medical appointments with a family medicine physician or internist are recommended for all patients who exhibit signs of an eating disorder. No matter the degree of psychological care they are receiving, all patients should have regular visits to monitor vital signs.

Treatments

Adaptations of evidence-based treatments are used for most treatment of eating disorders in the context of obesity (Figure 7–1). Leading evidence-based treatments, including family-based treatment (FBT), CBT, DBT, and interpersonal psychotherapy (IPT), are appropriate for eating disorders in the context of obesity. The overarching goal of treatment is the normalization of eating patterns. The most significant difference in treatment protocol from AN is that weight regain is not the primary outcome measure in treatment; clinicians should not expect patients to achieve premorbid weight, although weight gain is likely necessary in cases of food restriction for full return to health, including return or menses (Seetharaman et al. 2017). However, in cases of BN and BED in which the patient is obese, treatment may result in weight loss. Nevertheless, weight loss in these cases is not the primary treatment outcome.

Family-Based Treatment

FBT has a strong evidence base for younger patients who live at home with their families. Typically, the efficacy of FBT for AN is measured by weight gained through treatment, but this would not be the case for obese patients. The focus in this context would be to normalize eating patterns and pathology. In most cases this would include eating three meals and a couple of snacks daily. Given these goals, weight gain during treatment is expected. Regardless of weight, patients receiving FBT should be medically monitored to ensure stable vital signs.

One challenge of FBT in the context of obesity is tackling the family's existing habits. Children who are obese are 10–12 times more likely to have obese parents (Fuemmeler et al. 2013). With this in mind, clinicians providing FBT to an obese patient might have to adjust their approach to fit the family's

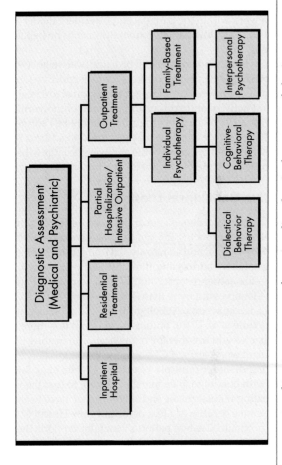

FIGURE 7–1. Assessment and treatment process for eating disorders in the context of obesity.

situation. The clinician will want to support the family in restoring healthy eating patterns but avoid being didactic or judgmental in the approach. For example, these families might historically eat out regularly or have inconsistent eating patterns themselves. The clinician might, in this situation, encourage the family to make adjustments when possible to support recovery and also support the family in learning about healthy eating in the context of their routine and environment. It is crucial to work within the parental empowerment model outlined in FBT and allow parents to make decisions on behalf of their family.

FBT has been adapted for use in pediatric overweight (without the presence of an eating disorder), which addresses some of this balance between providing information about healthy eating and activity and supporting parental empowerment (Loeb et al. 2015). As noted in the adaptation of FBT for pediatric overweight, the clinician may also need to address feelings of blame about the cause of the overweight status to begin with in order to move forward with healthy changes.

Cognitive-Behavioral Therapy

CBT for eating disorders is one of the most efficacious treatment methods for treating BN and BED, and it can be adapted for a patient with comorbid obesity. CBT targets eating disorder symptoms by addressing thoughts and behaviors. CBT for BED—the eating disorder that is most common in obese patients—is successful more than 50% of the time and also has a significant impact on psychological and psychosocial functioning (White et al. 2010). Studies have found it is more impactful than weight loss therapy or medication in treating BED, and patients who received CBT were still in remission from their eating disorder multiple years later (White et al. 2010). Patients with obesity may be initially resistant to (per the CBT model) eating regular meals and snacks if they have been restricting intake because of a fear of weight gain. However, the result of normalized eating patterns generally supports the reduction of binge eating and thus does not result in weight gain as patients fear.

Dialectical Behavior Therapy

DBT was conceptualized on the basis of research showing that patients use disordered eating behaviors as a coping mechanism for intense and seemingly intolerable emotional states (Linehan and Chen 2005). It is used widely in treating eating disorders—especially BED and BN—when patients have not responded to CBT. Patients with obesity may also benefit from the application of emotion regulation skills in managing stigma, guilt, and shame about their weight and eating behaviors.

Interpersonal Psychotherapy

IPT addresses interpersonal disturbances that affect eating behaviors and feelings about weight and shape. This treatment was initially developed to treat depression and was applied to the treatment of eating disorders in a transdiagnostic approach (Fairburn et al. 2015). Because the adaptation did not add many specific approaches for eating disorders specifically, IPT does not require much adaptation for patients with comorbid obesity and thus can be applied in a straightforward manner. Evidence suggests that CBT provides a faster and more successful treatment response, but IPT also has modest success over a more prolonged period (Fairburn et al. 2015).

Treatments Illustrated

Family-Based Treatment for Atypical Anorexia Nervosa in the Context of Obesity (see Case 1)

After Maria, the 17-year-old Mexican American female with atypical anorexia nervosa in the context of obesity whose case was described earlier, was hospitalized for orthostatic changes in heart rate, she and her family began FBT for atypical AN with an outpatient therapist.

Her parents were extremely confused about where to begin in feeding Maria. On the one hand, they were very concerned about her malnutrition and worried about her heart rate, which kept decreasing at each doctor visit. On the other hand, they noted that her previous weight status with a BMI of 37 made them fearful of returning to old patterns of eating. Maria's father struggles with weight-related type 2 diabetes himself, and he does not want that future for his daughter. Maria's family worked with their therapist to create a plan to support Maria in eating three meals and two snacks daily and incorporating a variety of types of foods in that plan. This meant, for example, challenging her recent fear of pasta, which had previously been a favorite food. Maria's weight was not low, so the family was focused on feeding for the purpose nourishing her body, which was clearly deprived, as evidenced by her fatigue and shift in heart rate rather than weight gain, per se. Because of the family's concerns about overweight and obesity, support in helping them understand the importance of a variety of foods and nutrients was important. Although they had heard about "healthy foods" focusing on vegetables and salads, they were encouraged to consider the health benefits of fats and carbohydrates, particularly for Maria's needs in nourishing her body back to health after a period of malnutrition.

Just as in FBT for AN, FBT for atypical AN is delivered in a series of three phases, with the first phase consisting of parents in charge of selecting what food, how much, and when to eat, as well as monitoring all meals and snacks to ensure they are eaten. One criterion for deciding when a family is ready to move to the second phase in FBT for AN relates to weight gain. However, in Maria's case, because she did not have an explicit goal of weight gain, the decision is influenced more by her response to the meals and snacks her parents select and the decrease in resistance to eating during meals. Phase 1 was challenging for Maria's parents. Despite her lack of low weight, her behaviors in response to monitored meals were very similar to those of patients with low-weight AN. During a meal session, when parents brought her spaghetti with meat sauce (a prior favorite meal), she refused to even hold the fork initially. As her mother supported her and helped her calm down, engaging in some relaxing conversation to try to distract her, placing a hand on her shoulder to help encourage her, Maria was able to take a small bite. This felt laborious and very slow to her parents, but they were encouraged and their efforts were validated by the small steps Maria took toward eating the pasta.

Over time, these efforts were more effective, and they were able to eat meals with less struggle, eventually ready to move toward more independence for Maria in phase 2 of treatment. This phase was also a challenge, as Maria was calm in eating what her parents served but still felt pressure to restrict and eat "healthy" foods on her own. Thus, initially her parents recommended that she start with portioning her meals with them so that they could ensure she was eating enough. As Maria felt more confident that her pattern of eating was not resulting in a return of obesity, she was also better able to engage in independent eating. Eventually, the family felt that eating was "back to normal," although they acknowledged that the family as a whole was eating more balanced meals with a variety of nutrients present. Phase 3 involved a focus on Maria's choice for an activity after the upcoming school dance, over which there was some disagreement between Maria and her parents.

Cognitive Behavior Therapy for Bulimia Nervosa in the Context of Obesity (see Case 2)

Jason's presentation with BED, coupled with his age (as described earlier), led his therapist to recommend CBT. They began working on food logs, where Jason would keep track of what foods he ate, when, where, and any context surrounding the eating. For example, he would note whether he considered the eating episode a binge or if there were any situations or precipitating circumstances involved in the eating. If he did engage in compensatory behaviors after eating, he was instructed to make note of that, too, although in Jason's case, he did not have any of these behaviors to report. An additional part of the instruction was to engage in regular eating patterns. This meant ensuring that there was no food restriction and that he was eating every 3–4 hours. Because of Jason's weight and his history of being overweight since childhood, he initially expressed some concern about food monitoring. He feared that he would eat too much. He was especially concerned about eating every 3–4 hours, as that would include at least some snacks, which he feared would become binge episodes. He agreed to the plan, however, because the therapist encouraged him to be open-minded and use the logs as a learning tool to identify patterns in his eating behaviors.

Initially, Jason noticed a pattern in his logs: he was more likely to engage in binge eating on days when he ate what he considered "unhealthy" foods, such as burgers or pastas. If he stuck with meals that were lower in fat content, such as quinoa with fish and vegetables or salad with grilled chicken and a light vinaigrette dressing, he was less likely to engage in binge eating. Upon exploring this pattern, he initially thought that sticking with the "healthy" foods would prevent binge eating. With direction from the therapist, he was able to observe a larger pattern beyond the single day. He noted that "good days" were often followed by "bad days," which could be a direct response to the food rules. He noted feeling strong cravings for burgers or pastas on the "bad days" and then feeling frustrated with himself for his choice of food. He ended up throwing out all attempts at restraint after he ate something "unhealthy" because of this frustration, which then resulted in binge eating. This pattern suggested that there was nothing inherently wrong with eating the burgers or pastas that led to binge eating, but rather his response to those choices. He was also able to identify the connection between his low-fat eating on "good days" and his subsequent craving for fats and carbohydrates on the following days. His therapist suggested an experiment of incorporating more fats and carbohydrates into his meals on the "good days" to see how that impacted his cravings. Furthermore, they worked together to address his thoughts about "unhealthy" foods in attempt to reframe them as an important part of a balanced diet when eaten in moderation. Thus, the use of behavior change—as well as challenging thoughts about eating patterns—could reduce the occurrence of binge eating. Although this was easy to talk about during therapy, and hard to implement, over time Jason found that this new approach to his diet was more acceptable. He was anxious about gaining weight in response to allowing himself to eat the "unhealthy" foods but eventually was able to see how the result of incorporating those foods into his diet in moderation reduced the out-of-control intake when he attempted to cut them out of his diet.

Dialectical Behavior Therapy for Binge-Eating Disorder in the Context of Obesity (see Case 3)

After an initial trial of CBT to regulate eating patterns disrupted by her BN (as described earlier), Monica and her therapist realized that a lingering precipitant for her binge eating that was not addressed adequately in CBT was her difficulty managing her emotions. Despite stopping her calorie limit and balancing her overall food intake, Monica was still engaging in binge eating on "comfort foods" when she was upset, particularly when she was missing home. Thus, her therapist suggested trying DBT. They began working on mindfulness, a core skill utilized through DBT, and also introduced diary cards to monitor the use of DBT skills. Over the course of treatment, Monica was able to utilize distress tolerance and emotion regulation skills to better manage her emotional response. Importantly, she also benefited from interpersonal effectiveness skills, as many of her emotional reactions were based on difficult interpersonal experiences. Applying these skills, along with a firm commitment to stop engaging in binge eating and purging behaviors through therapy, allowed her to find more adaptive solutions. She ended up losing a bit of weight because of the reduction in binge eating and the regulated eating pattern she had already established when completing CBT prior to engaging in DBT.

Common Outcomes and Complications

- Resistance to treatment due to fear of weight gain, denial of illness, or other reason

    - These patients are already overweight or obese, so they may be especially resistant to any weight gain during treatment. They might use their weight to deny their illness, claiming that one cannot have an eating disorder and also be overweight.

- Skepticism from other healthcare professionals

    - The aim is for the entire treatment team to be aligned on the patient's goals. It is possible, however, due to the misconceptions about eating disorders previously discussed, that other professionals might question the patient's course of treatment. If this happens, the clinician should explain the basis for the diagnosis and why treatment is imperative.

- Development of a different eating disorder during treatment

    - Sometimes patients develop different eating disorder symptoms in response to treatment. For example, this might happen with a patient with atypical anorexia nervosa who gains weight during recovery. To combat weight gain, he or she might start to purge or engage in other compensatory behaviors. Clinicians should watch for other symptoms and address them as soon as they arise.

Resources and Further Reading

Training Resources

CBT: Oxford Cognitive Therapy Centre: https://www.octc.co.uk/training

FBT: Training Institute for Child and Adolescent Eating Disorders: http://train2treat4ed.com

DBT: Behavioral Tech: https://behavioraltech.org

Fairburn CG: Cognitive Behavioral Therapy and Eating Disorders. New York, Guilford, 2008

Lock J, Le Grange D: Treatment Manual for Anorexia Nervosa: A Family Based Approach, 2nd Edition. New York, Guilford, 2013

Murphy R, Straebler S, Cooper Z, et al: Interpersonal psychotherapy (IPT) for the treatment of eating disorders, in Evidence Based Treatments for Eating Disorders. Edited by Dancyger IF, Fornari V. New York, Nova, 2009, pp 257–275

Safer DL, Telch CF, Chen EY: Dialectical Behavior Therapy for Binge Eating and Bulimia. New York, Guilford, 2009

STOP Obesity Alliance: Why Weight? A Guide to Discussing Obesity and Health With Your Patients, 2014. Available at: http://whyweightguide.org.

Tanofsky-Kraft M, Shomaker L, Young J, et al: Interpersonal psychotherapy for eating disorders and the prevention of excess weight gain, in Casebook of Evidence-Based Treatments for Eating Disorders. Edited by Thompson-Brenner H. New York, Guilford, 2015, pp 195–219

Other Resources

The Body Positive: www.thebodypositive.org
Health at Every Size: haescommunity.com
National Eating Disorders Association: www.nationaleatingdisorders.org
Stop Obesity Alliance: whyweightguide.org

Further Reading

Bacon L: Healthy at Every Size: The Surprising Truth About Your Weight. Dallas, TX, Benbella Books, 2010

Fairburn CG, Brownell KD: Eating Disorders and Obesity: A Comprehensive Handbook, 2nd Edition. New York, Guilford, 2005

Golden NH, Schneider M, Wood C, et al: Preventing eating disorders and obesity in adolescents. Pediatrics 138(3):e1–e10, 2016

Sim LA, Lebow J, Billings M: Eating disorders in adolescents with a history of obesity. Pediatrics 132(4):e1026–1030, 2013

References

Agras WS, Walsh T, Fairburn CG, et al: A multicenter comparison of cognitive-behavioral therapy and interpersonal psychotherapy for bulimia nervosa. Arch Gen Psychiatry 57(5):459–466, 2000 10807486

Alexander J, Goldschmidt A, Le Grange D: A Clinician's Guide to Binge Eating Disorder. Abingdon, United Kingdom, Routledge, 2013

American Psychiatric Association: Diagnostic and Statistical Manual of Mental Disorders, 5th Edition. Arlington, VA, American Psychiatric Association, 2013

Andreyeva T, Puhl RM, Brownell KD: Changes in perceived weight discrimination among Americans, 1995–1996 through 2004–2006. Obesity (Silver Spring) 16(5):1129–1134, 2008 18356847

Cassin SE, von Ranson KM: Personality and eating disorders: a decade in review. Clin Psychol Rev 25(7):895–916, 2005 16099563

Citrome L: Binge-eating disorder and comorbid conditions: differential diagnosis and implications for treatment. J Clin Psychiatry 78(suppl 1):9–13, 2017 28125173

Fairburn CG, Stice E, Cooper Z, et al: Understanding persistence in bulimia nervosa: a 5-year naturalistic study. J Consult Clin Psychol 71(1):103–109, 2003 12602430

Fairburn CG, Cooper Z, Shafran R: Enhanced cognitive behavioral therapy for eating disorders ("CBT-E"), in Cognitive Behavior Therapy and Eating Disorders. New York, Guilford, 2008, pp 23–34

Fairburn CG, Bailey-Straebler S, Basden S, et al: A transdiagnostic comparison of enhanced cognitive behaviour therapy (CBT-E) and interpersonal psychotherapy in the treatment of eating disorders. Behav Res Ther 70(suppl C):64–71, 2015 26000757

Faulconbridge LF, Bechtel CF: Depression and disordered eating in the obese person. Curr Obes Rep 3(1):127–136, 2014 24678445

Frisch MJ, Herzog DB, Franko DL: Residential treatment for eating disorders. Int J Eat Disord 39(5):434–442, 2006 16528698

Fuemmeler BF, Lovelady CA, Zucker NL, et al: Parental obesity moderates the relationship between childhood appetitive traits and weight. Obesity (Silver Spring) 21(4):815–823, 2013 23712985

Holderness CC, Brooks-Gunn J, Warren MP: Co-morbidity of eating disorders and substance abuse review of the literature. Int J Eat Disord 16(1):1–34, 1994 7920577

Hruby A, Hu FB: The epidemiology of obesity: a big picture. Pharmacoeconomics 33(7):673–689, 2015 25471927

Kaye WH, Bulik CM, Thornton L, et al: Comorbidity of anxiety disorders with anorexia and bulimia nervosa. Am J Psychiatry 161(12):2215–2221, 2004 15569892

Lavie CJ, Milani RV, Ventura HO: Obesity and cardiovascular disease: risk factor, paradox, and impact of weight loss. J Am Coll Cardiol 53(21):1925–1932, 2009 19460605

Le Grange D, Lock J, Agras WS, et al: Randomized clinical trial of family based treatment and cognitive-behavioral therapy for adolescent bulimia nervosa. J Am Acad Child Adolesc Psychiatry 54(11):886–894, 2015 26506579

Linehan MM, Chen EY: Dialectical behavior therapy for eating disorders, in Encyclopedia of Cognitive Behavior Therapy. Springer, Boston, MA, 2005, pp 168–171

Loeb KL, Doyle AC, Anderson K, et al: Family based treatment for child and adolescent overweight and obesity, in Family Therapy for Adolescent Eating and Weight Disorders: New Applications. Edited by Loeb KL, Le Grange D, Lock J. New York, Routledge, 2015, pp 177–229

Luppino FS, de Wit LM, Bouvy PF, et al: Overweight, obesity, and depression: a systematic review and meta-analysis of longitudinal studies. Arch Gen Psychiatry 67(3):220–229, 2010 20194822

Puhl R, Suh Y: Stigma and eating and weight disorders. Curr Psychiatry Rep 17(3):552, 2015 25652251

Re RN: Obesity-related hypertension. Ochsner J 9(3):133–136, 2009 21603428

Safer DL, Telch CF, Agras WS: Dialectical behavior therapy for bulimia nervosa. Am J Psychiatry 158(4):632–634, 2001 11282700

Seetharaman S, Golden NH, Halpern-Felsher B, et al: Effect of a prior history of overweight on return of menses in adolescents with eating disorders. J Adolesc Health 60(4):469–471, 2017 27998699

Thornton LM, Mazzeo SE, Bulik CM: The heritability of eating disorders: methods and current findings. Curr Top Behav Neurosci 6:141–156, 2011 21243474

White MA, Grilo CM, O'Malley SS, et al: Clinical case discussion: binge eating disorder, obesity and tobacco smoking. J Addict Med 4(1):11–19, 2010 20436923

Index

Page numbers printed in **boldface** *type refer to tables or figures.*